NATIONAL ACADEMIES

Sciences
Engineering
Medicine

NATIONAL ACADEMIES PRESS
Washington, DC

Substance Misuse Programs in Commercial Aviation

Safety First

Richard G. Frank, Dylan Rebstock, and Melissa Welch-Ross, *Editors*

Committee on the Study and Recommendations on the HIMS, FADAP, and Other Drug and Alcohol Programs within the USDOT

Board on Behavioral, Cognitive, and Sensory Sciences

Division of Behavioral and Social Sciences and Education

Transportation Research Board

Health and Medicine Division

Consensus Study Report

NATIONAL ACADEMIES PRESS 500 Fifth Street, NW Washington, DC 20001

This activity was supported by a contract between the National Academy of Sciences and the Federal Aviation Administration (#693KA9-22-T-00002). Any opinions, findings, conclusions, or recommendations expressed in this publication do not necessarily reflect the views of any organization or agency that provided support for the project.

International Standard Book Number-13: 978-0-309-70278-2
International Standard Book Number-10: 0-309-70278-X
Digital Object Identifier: https://doi.org/10.17226/27025
Library of Congress Control Number: 2023944913

This publication is available from the National Academies Press, 500 Fifth Street, NW, Keck 360, Washington, DC 20001; (800) 624-6242 or (202) 334-3313; http://www.nap.edu.

Suggested citation: National Academies of Sciences, Engineering, and Medicine. 2023. *Substance Misuse Programs in Commercial Aviation: Safety First.* Washington, DC: The National Academies Press. https://doi.org/10.17226/27025.

The **National Academy of Sciences** was established in 1863 by an Act of Congress, signed by President Lincoln, as a private, nongovernmental institution to advise the nation on issues related to science and technology. Members are elected by their peers for outstanding contributions to research. Dr. Marcia McNutt is president.

The **National Academy of Engineering** was established in 1964 under the charter of the National Academy of Sciences to bring the practices of engineering to advising the nation. Members are elected by their peers for extraordinary contributions to engineering. Dr. John L. Anderson is president.

The **National Academy of Medicine** (formerly the Institute of Medicine) was established in 1970 under the charter of the National Academy of Sciences to advise the nation on medical and health issues. Members are elected by their peers for distinguished contributions to medicine and health. Dr. Victor J. Dzau is president.

The three Academies work together as the **National Academies of Sciences, Engineering, and Medicine** to provide independent, objective analysis and advice to the nation and conduct other activities to solve complex problems and inform public policy decisions. The National Academies also encourage education and research, recognize outstanding contributions to knowledge, and increase public understanding in matters of science, engineering, and medicine.

Learn more about the National Academies of Sciences, Engineering, and Medicine at **www.nationalacademies.org**.

Reviewers

This Consensus Study Report was reviewed in draft form by individuals chosen for their diverse perspectives and technical expertise. The purpose of this independent review is to provide candid and critical comments that will assist the National Academies of Sciences, Engineering, and Medicine in making each published report as sound as possible and to ensure that it meets the institutional standards for quality, objectivity, evidence, and responsiveness to the study charge. The review comments and draft manuscript remain confidential to protect the integrity of the deliberative process.

We thank the following individuals for their review of this report:

RICHARD N. ASLIN, Yale University
JONATHAN P. CAULKINS, Carnegie Mellon University
NICOLE ENNIS, Florida State University
CHRISTIAN HOPFER, University of Colorado Anschutz Medical Campus
DENNIS McCARTY, Oregon Health & State University
JOSIAH D. RICH, Miriam Hospital, Brown University
PAUL M. ROMAN, University of Georgia
CHRISTINE TIMKO, U.S. Department of Veterans Affairs
EUGENIA VASQUEZ, University of Colorado

Although the reviewers listed above provided many constructive comments and suggestions, they were not asked to endorse the conclusions or recommendations of this report nor did they see the final draft before its release. The review of this report was overseen by **ROBERT WALLACE,**

University of Iowa, and **HORTENSIA AMARO,** Florida International University. They were responsible for making certain that an independent examination of this report was carried out in accordance with the standards of the National Academies and that all review comments were carefully considered. Responsibility for the final content rests entirely with the authoring committee and the National Academies.

Acknowledgments

This report reflects contributions from a number of individuals and groups. The committee takes this opportunity to recognize those who so generously gave their time and expertise to inform its deliberations.

To begin, the committee would like to thank the Federal Aviation Administration and the Office of Senator Jeanne Shaheen for their sponsorship, guidance, and support of this study.

The committee greatly benefited from the opportunity for discussion with individuals who attended and presented at the open session meetings or provided written testimony: Kip Bowen, David Fielding, Heather Healy, Suzanne Kalfus, Andrew LeBovidge, Rick Mahoney, Tom McLellan, Pat Moy, Billy Petersen, Sarah Polk, Jerry Powers, Bryan Price, Iyon Rosario, Quay Snyder, David St. Helaire, and Nora Volkow. The committee thanks these individuals for their time and the candid perspectives they provided.

The committee could not have done its work without the support and guidance provided by the National Academies of Sciences, Engineering, and Medicine project staff: Dylan Rebstock, Study Director; Melissa Welch-Ross, Senior Program Officer; Lyle Carrera, Research Associate; and Jacqueline L. Cole, Senior Program Assistant. We appreciate Patrick Burke for his financial assistance on this project and gratefully acknowledge Daniel J. Weiss of the National Academies' Board on Behavioral, Cognitive, and Sensory Sciences for his guidance.

Many other staff within the National Academies provided support to this project in various ways. The committee would like to thank Samantha Chao, Connie Citro, Chris King, Sandy McDermin, Tom Menzies, Sharyl

Nass, Kirsten Sampson Snyder, and Jeanne Rivard for their expertise and support throughout the life cycle of this research study and report.

This committee is grateful to the research assistants and commissioned paper authors who generously contributed to this body of work: Heather Belanger, Anne Marie Houppert, Gary Kay, Christopher Lao-Scott, Cara Nordberg, and Jennifer Wisdom.

In addition to the contributions above, a great number of stakeholders offered resources, expertise, and insight to support the committee's work.

Contents

Appendixes

Boxes, Figures, and Tables

TABLES

Acronyms and Abbreviations

AA	Alcoholics Anonymous
AFA-CWA	Association of Flight Attendants-CWA
ALPA	Air Line Pilots Association, International
AME	aviation medical examiner
ASAM	American Society of Addiction Medicine
CDLs	commercial driving licenses
CFR	Code of Federal Regulations
CMVs	commercial motor vehicles
DAC	drug and alcohol counselor
DOT	U.S. Department of Transportation
DSM-5	*Diagnostic and Statistical Manual of Mental Disorders, Fifth Edition*
DSM-5-TR	Text Revision of the *Diagnostic and Statistical Manual of Mental Disorders, Fifth Edition*
DUI	driving under the influence
EAP	Employee Assistance Program
FAA	Federal Aviation Administration
FADAP	Flight Attendant Drug and Alcohol Program
FMCSA	Federal Motor Carrier Safety Administration

FRA	Federal Railroad Administration
FTA	Federal Transit Administration
HHS	U.S. Department of Health and Human Services
HIMS	Human Intervention and Motivational Study
HIMS AME	Human Intervention and Motivational Study-trained aviation medical examiner
IOP	intensive outpatient program
LOS	length of stay
MAT	medication-assisted treatment
MAUD	medications for alcohol use disorder
MHGs	mutual help groups
MOUD	medications for opioid use disorder
NA	Narcotics Anonymous
NIAAA	National Institute on Alcohol Abuse and Alcoholism
NTSB	National Transportation Safety Board
OTC	over-the-counter
OTP	opioid treatment program
P&P	[HIMS-trained] psychiatrist and neuropsychologist
PHPs	Physician Health Programs
ROI	release of information
SAMHSA	Substance Abuse and Mental Health Services Administration
SAP	substance abuse professional
SBIRT	screening, brief intervention, and referral to treatment
WHO	World Health Organization
XR-naltrexone	extended-release injectable naltrexone

Summary

Substance use disorders are prevalent in the United States. The National Institutes of Health define a substance use disorder as "a treatable mental disorder that affects a person's brain and behavior, leading to their inability to control their use of substances like legal or illegal drugs, alcohol, or [prescription] medications." (National Institute of Mental Health, n.d.). National estimates suggest that about 15 percent of the population age 18 and older has a substance use disorder, more than two-thirds of them an alcohol use disorder (SAMHSA, 2021). For the purposes of this report, the committee defined *substance misuse*[1] as substance use that is problematic from a health, policy, or regulatory perspective, even when it might not meet the diagnostic threshold of a substance use disorder. Substance misuse also includes using substances in inappropriate settings, such as the workplace, or in high doses (McLellan, 2017). The prevalence rate of substance misuse among pilots and flight attendants is uncertain, due to the limited validated data that are available. The general view held both in the literature (Modell & Mountz, 1990; Porges, 2013) and by the Federal Aviation Administration (FAA)[2,3] is that the prevalence rate potentially lies in the

---

[1]Although not a universally adopted term, the committee chose to follow the precedent of the Department of Health and Human Services, the Centers for Disease Control and Prevention, and the Surgeon General in using "substance misuse" in this report to describe a broad spectrum of substance use that could be considered problematic from a policy or regulatory perspective despite not meeting the diagnostic threshold of a substance use disorder.

[2]Flight Attendant Drug and Alcohol Program (FADAP) staff response to the Committee-issued questionnaire, August 2022.

[3]HIMS staff response to the Committee-issued questionnaire, August 2022.

range of 8 to 15 percent, which is roughly comparable to the range in the general population.

The job of commercial airline pilots is not like other jobs. Pilots are entrusted with people's lives while operating a complex machine that engages all neurocognitive domains. Pilots must be prepared to respond rapidly, both cognitively and physically, to altered circumstances in jet aircraft traveling at high speeds in an environment susceptible to rapid change. Flight attendants too must be prepared to respond quickly and effectively in high pressure situations that can change abruptly.

Ensuring that pilots and flight attendants who need treatment for substance misuse are excused from their duties to receive effective treatment is critical for both aviation safety and the health and well-being of pilots. That requires commitment from the government, the employer, the airlines, and the affected individuals. Substance misuse can have a wide range of negative consequences on a person's life, adversely affecting physical and mental health, relationships, finances, and careers. For many reasons, it is in the public interest to help people obtain effective treatment for their substance misuse and return to work. Otherwise, society faces safety risks and the potential loss of highly skilled pilots and trained flight attendants from the commercial airline workforce.

Established in 1974, the Human Intervention and Motivational Study (HIMS) is a program that coordinates the identification, treatment, return to work, and monitoring of pilots who misuse substances. Similarly, the FADAP, created in 2010, supports flight attendants who misuse substances or have a substance use disorder. Endorsed by the FAA, airlines, and employee unions, both programs seek to ensure aviation safety and preserve the careers of these critical airline workers.

This study, which was sponsored by the FAA in response to a congressional mandate, reviews available evidence and program information on HIMS and FADAP. When it began, a key goal of the study was to identify policies and practices from the two programs that could be relevant and helpful to improving the drug and alcohol programs of other transportation modes. It was also understood, however, that the review could surface needed improvements in HIMS and FADAP, or perhaps point to areas where assessments and evaluations need to be strengthened to improve the effectiveness of the two programs. See Box S-1 for the complete statement of task.

STUDY APPROACH

To conduct the study, the National Academies of Sciences, Engineering, and Medicine appointed a 12-member committee consisting of experts in program evaluation, state regulation of safety-related professions, health economics, and the clinical disciplines (psychiatry and psychology) relevant

---

BOX S-1
Project Statement of Task

Pursuant to Section 554 of the FAA Reauthorization Act of 2018, the National Academies of Sciences, Engineering, and Medicine will conduct a consensus study to:

- Identify relevant drug and alcohol programs within U.S. Department of Transportation (DOT) and its modal administrations, and similar industries and sectors, beyond HIMS and FADAP;
- Review available assessments and evaluation information on the HIMS, FADAP, and any other identified drug and alcohol programs to identify:
  - Best policies and practices within existing programs; and
  - Best practices for prevention, early intervention, and return to work specifically around prescription medication abuse, with an emphasis on employee use of opioids; and
  - To the extent justified by the evidence, provide recommendations to the FAA and other modal administrations within the DOT on how to implement programs, or change existing programs, that seek to help transportation workers get treatment for drug and alcohol abuse and return to work.

The committee will deliver a report to FAA and the appropriate committees of Congress on the study, including findings, conclusions, and recommendations.

---

to the evaluation and treatment of people with substance use disorders in the airline workforce and other safety-sensitive occupations. At the study outset, the committee assembled information on the histories of the programs and their methods. The committee learned that prior to 1974, the FAA lacked a rehabilitative program to encourage pilots to seek help with recovery and remission to return to work safely. With a grant from the National Institute on Alcohol Abuse and Alcoholism, the Air Line Pilots Association, International (ALPA), in cooperation with the FAA and airlines, created HIMS as a prototype occupational substance use program for pilots. HIMS was intended to provide a comprehensive approach to rehabilitation and recovery by emphasizing identification of pilots misusing substances, diagnostic assessment, treatment, continuing care, monitoring, and relapse assistance. FADAP was created for flight attendants after HIMS had been in place for pilots for more than 35 years.

After gathering information about the HIMS and FADAP histories and methods, the committee reviewed presentations and reports prepared by HIMS and FADAP administrators to assess program outcomes and determine the content of program activities. To supplement and independently assess the reports from the programs, the committee requested access to HIMS and FADAP databases that included more detailed information on treatment and outcomes. The committee intended to conduct analyses that would provide a more complete and detailed description of the work and outcomes produced by the programs with the aid of a consultant hired for the study. In order to obtain more qualitative information on the, lived experiences (a "Call for Perspectives") of pilots and flight attendants, some of whom may have participated in the programs, the committee developed a tool for eliciting such information. Committee members and staff also attended annual meetings of the two programs, met with program administrators and stakeholders, and arranged to interview a small group of participants to gain additional, first-hand qualitative information about the programs.

In order to put the processes and approaches of the HIMS and FADAP in context, the committee reviewed the robust literature that has emerged over the past few decades on methods to treat and support people who have misuse substances and have substance use disorders. In reviewing this literature and consulting experts in substance use disorder treatment, the committee documented the changes occurring in treatment based on the disease model of addiction. The methods employed by HIMS and FADAP could thus be compared with the state of the clinical science and practice for screening, assessing, and treating professionals with substance use disorders in safety-sensitive occupations. Additionally, the committee focused on examining the evidence base behind alcohol use disorder treatment because alcohol was the most frequent substance being misused in the aviation industry. The same general principles (to varying degrees) apply to all substances with addiction potential, including misused prescription drugs and opioids.

In pursuing this study plan the committee encountered several challenges, particularly with respect to HIMS. Notably, the committee's effort to undertake an independent analysis of the workings of HIMS was hindered by a lack of access to program records and testimony from pilots on their lived experience. Repeated requests to share de-identified program outcome data with one professional statistician, even with assurances of confidentiality and under the oversight of the National Academies' Institutional Review Board, were denied by HIMS administrators. Other efforts to ensure protection of the data, including conduct of the analysis by HIMS staff, were rebuffed. Moreover, the committee never received indications that ALPA-HIMS widely circulated the committee's "Call for Perspectives" tool for gathering lived experiences among pilots, foreclosing this assessment mechanism.[4] The result was that the committee obtained just nine responses from pilots. The administrators of FADAP, by comparison, circulated the "Call for Perspectives" to flight attendants and garnered more than 1,000 responses. The committee was successful in holding follow-on qualitative interviews with flight attendants. In contrast, the committee did not receive information on meaningful participation by pilots in this phase of the study. The committee invited pilots to the study's sole public workshop, but the invited pilots were advised not to participate after having discussions with their union representatives and airline senior staff. In the absence of a range of perspectives from pilots who had participated in HIMS, the committee could obtain the views of only two pilots, both ALPA members with HIMS leadership positions either at the national or airline level. In the case of FADAP only, the committee was able to commission the work of an independent consultant to help analyze program records, flight attendant survey results, and the qualitative interviews of several flight attendants who had either participated in FADAP directly or provided insights into the state of substance use within the profession. Unfortunately, the FADAP data were an incomplete reflection of the population of flight attendants, and a large share of participants were lost to follow-up and therefore outcome data were incomplete.

Unable to fully execute its original study plan, the committee was nevertheless able to reach a number of conclusions about the two programs, leading to recommendations on how to increase the reach and effectiveness of the two programs. These recommendations are summarized next.[5]

SUMMARY OF CONCLUSIONS AND RECOMMENDATIONS

The committee sought to understand the two programs' efforts on prevention and treatment by seeking answers to three questions: (1) How are pilots and flight attendants that misuse substances identified? (2) How do pilots and flight attendants that misuse substances and need treatment get engaged with treatment? and (3) How are flight attendants and pilots in need of follow-up care directed to appropriate and effective providers of care?

Three overarching observations informed the committee's recommendations.

First, the committee was cognizant of the precarious balance in

---

[4]After a prepublication version of the report was provided to the FAA, text was changed here and throughout the report to reflect that what was previously termed a survey was in fact a "Call for Perspectives."

[5]For an overview of each chapter and appendix, see Chapter 1.

commercial aviation between ensuring public safety and honoring the obligation to help employees in safety-sensitive positions receive the treatment to address their misuse of substances. The primary role and responsibility of the FAA is public safety, and thus it is reasonable for it to mandate more restrictive standards for substance misuse among its workers than are mandated for the general population. The committee found areas where the treatment arranged by HIMS and FADAP was not consistent with treatments grounded in evidence-based science where it appears possible to realize better outcomes while minimizing risk to the public. These areas include approaches to diagnosis and case identification, removal of barriers to early help-seeking and access to treatment, allowances and encouragement for individualized treatment, and use of evidence-based criteria in the selection of treatment programs.

Second, the implementation of substance misuse programs for pilots and flight attendants is highly decentralized, creating challenges for determining how to take the recommended actions that would align the programs with evidence-based practices.

Third, the implementation of effective programs necessarily depends on the ability to assess and monitor practices and outcomes for appropriate management and oversight. As described in Chapter 1, the committee experienced challenges with accessing data about the programs. Based on its review of the publicly reported data and the program data received from FADAP, the committee also developed concerns about the type and quality of data available to the FAA and the Congress that those bodies need to fulfill their management and oversight roles.

The committee's detailed conclusions and recommendations can be found in Chapter 6.

Recommendation 1: The Federal Aviation Administration should revise sections of the Code of Federal Regulations (CFR), especially 14 CFR Part 67 (Medical Standards and Certification), to align, to the extent reasonable in the aviation setting, with the most current evidence-based diagnostic approaches for substance use disorders that consider illness severity and lead to more personalized treatment.

Recommendation 2: The Federal Aviation Administration should ensure that mandated annual physical exams (e.g., aviation medical examiner examination) for all safety-sensitive professions that require screening for substance misuse use tools that are validated for the population and setting.

Recommendation 3: While employment termination is a legitimate outcome if return-to-work policies are not met, the Federal Aviation

Administration should ensure that airlines identify and remove features of their workplace substance misuse policies and procedures that are likely barriers to early identification and treatment, such as disclosures that are not likely related to performance in a safety-sensitive position, and consider opportunities to promote more fully early identification and treatment.

Recommendation 4: Commercial airline carriers should ensure affordable access for mental health and substance misuse related services for pilots and flight attendants consistent with the Mental Health Parity and Addiction Equity Act.

Recommendation 5: Administrators of both the Human Intervention and Motivational Study and the Flight Attendant Drug and Alcohol Program, with the support of the Federal Aviation Administration, should encourage and support individualized treatment and continuing care programs based on the severity of the individual pilot's or flight attendant's substance misuse and that person's preferences.

Recommendation 6: National Human Intervention Motivational Study (HIMS) and Flight Attendant Drug and Alcohol Program (FADAP) organizations should provide clear criteria that follow from evidence on effective treatment for the selection and approval of treatment settings to which each airline's HIMS/FADAP can make referrals.

Recommendation 7: In the service of effective oversight and continuous improvement of the Human Intervention Motivational Study (HIMS) and based on our analysis of the Flight Attendant Drug and Alcohol Program (FADAP) database, the Federal Aviation Administration (FAA) should require that FADAP collect and maintain more reliable and complete data. Based on the lack of independent analysis of the HIMS database, the FAA should require that HIMS collect and maintain reliable and complete data. Data collected for both programs should at minimum include: the number of pilots and flight attendants who contact them, the number of pilots and flight attendants referred for treatment, patterns and components of treatment, and long-term post-treatment outcomes.

1

Introduction

The problem of substance use disorders in the United States is profound. National estimates indicate that 15.4 percent of the U.S. adult population had a substance use disorder during 2020 (Substance Abuse and Mental Health Services Administration [SAMHSA], 2021). Of that total, the most prevalent condition was alcohol use disorders, although opioid use continues to be a major national concern. The National Institutes of Health defines a substance use disorder as "a treatable mental disorder that affects a person's brain and behavior, leading to their inability to control their use of substances like legal or illegal drugs, alcohol, or [prescription] medications" (National Institute of Mental Health, n.d.). For the purposes of this report, the committee defined substance misuse as substance use that is problematic from a health, policy, or regulatory perspective, regardless of whether such use meets the diagnostic threshold of a substance use disorder. Substance misuse also includes using substances in inappropriate settings, such as the workplace, or in high doses (McLellan, 2017).[1]

The negative consequences of substance use disorder or misuse can affect virtually all aspects of a person's life: physical and mental health, cognitive ability, relationships, finances, and career. The physical health effects can include sleep difficulties, liver disease, heart disease, cancer,

---

[1]While not a universally adopted term, the committee chose to follow the precedent of the Department of Health and Human Services (HHS), the Centers for Disease Control, and the Surgeon General in using "substance misuse" in this report to describe the broad spectrum of problematic substance use from a policy/regulatory perspective that might not rise to the diagnostic threshold of a substance use disorder.

respiratory issues, and even death. Acute intoxication slows reaction times and causes impairments in balance, motor skills, and judgement. The long-term effects of substance use disorder can include cognitive and neurological impairment. In addition to the above effects, clinical substance use disorders can compromise social functioning, leading to isolation, conflict, and broken trust in relationships. They also affect productivity, as evidenced by increases in sick days at work and job loss. Finally, substance misuse is associated with failure to meet financial responsibilities such as mortgage payments.

The cognitive and neurological impacts of alcohol use disorder are varied and wide-ranging. Some of the more common effects include memory impairment, difficulty with abstract thinking, disinhibition, and difficulty with decision-making (Bates et al., 2013; Evert & Oscar-Berman, 1995; Nixon, 1995). Long-term heavy use of alcohol can lead to permanent changes in the brain, including damage to the hippocampus and other areas associated with memory and learning (Modell & Mountz, 1990). In people without acquired tolerance, impairments for complex skills can start to occur at blood alcohol levels of 0.025 percent. Alcohol doses at the 0.05 percent level have been shown to affect gross motor control and orientation. In addition to cognitive effects, alcohol use disorder can cause neurological effects, such as seizures, tremors, and impaired coordination (Modell & Mountz, 1990).

Because substance use disorders can affect people's work in all professions and jobs, there is reasonable concern about workers in transportation, especially in aviation, given the responsibilities those workers hold for the lives of others. While there is little validated data for this population, it has been suggested that the prevalence rate of substance use disorders for pilots may be similar to that of the general population (Porges, 2013). With this as context, in 1974 the Human Intervention Motivational Study (HIMS) began as a program to support pilots with a grant to the Air Line Pilots Association, International (ALPA) from the National Institute on Alcohol Abuse and Alcoholism. The Flight Attendant Drug and Alcohol Program (FADAP) was then initiated in 2010 to provide guidance and resources for flight attendants. Available data from these programs, although limited, confirm alcohol as the substance misused most often among program participants; greater than 80 percent of people treated under FADAP were suffering from alcohol use disorder. Similarly, limited data from HIMS show that greater than 90 percent of the pilots participating in HIMS had an alcohol use disorder. Regarding the use of stimulants (methamphetamines and cocaine), the rates were roughly 16 percent in FADAP and about 4 percent in HIMS. A very small share (2% or less) of pilots and flight attendants misused opioids. Nevertheless, the limited data available from aviation events provide reason for concern about the potential impacts of prescription medication or illicit opioid misuse, particularly when combined with an opioid epidemic that continues in the general population of the United States.[2]

Currently the Bureau of Labor Statistics estimates that 48,750 active commercial pilots are employed by airlines (Bureau of Labor Statistics [BLS], 2022a) and 108,480 flight attendants are employed by the airline industry (BLS, 2022b). Given the national substance use disorder prevalence rates of 13 to 15 percent, one might expect that between 6,300 and 7,300 pilots would meet diagnostic criteria annually and that a considerably larger number could engage in substance misuse that does not meet diagnostic thresholds. Likewise, these data suggest that between 14,100 and 16,200 flight attendants could meet criteria of a diagnosable substance use disorder.

The Federal Aviation Administration (FAA) Reauthorization Act of 2018 required the secretary of the U.S. Department of Transportation (DOT) to enter into an agreement with the National Academies of Sciences, Engineering, and Medicine to conduct a study on HIMS and FADAP and other DOT drug and alcohol programs: see Box 1-1 for the complete statement of task.

Within the National Academies, three units participated in the study: the Board on Behavioral, Cognitive, and Sensory Sciences in the Division of Behavioral and Social Sciences and Education; the Transportation Research Board; and the Health and Medicine Division. The committee appointed to carry out the study was composed of experts with the range of skills and backgrounds necessary to assess the workings of programs such as FADAP and HIMS, including psychiatrists and psychologists who focus on the treatment of people with substance use disorders in safety-sensitive occupations, psychologists who regularly evaluate pilots participating in HIMS, evaluation specialists, professionals who oversee state regulation of safety-related professions involving the transportation industry, and health economists.

---

[2]Concerns over the impact of substance misuse have been heightened by FAA investigations of civil aviation crashes that show a strong association of such events with evidence of substance misuse. The prevalence of potentially impairing substance use in aviation has frequently been measured by toxicology reports of pilots who died in aviation accidents. For example, in the area of drug use, data from the FAA Civil Aerospace Medical Institute's Forensic Sciences Laboratory toxicology database and the National Transportation Safety Board's aviation accident database were used to examine trends in the prevalence of over-the-counter, prescription, and illicit drug use by pilots during the years 1990–2012, and during follow-up years, 2013–2017. Findings of the two analyses showed increasing trends in the proportions of study pilots testing positive for at least one drug categorized as potentially impairing, used to treat a potentially impairing condition, or as a controlled substance (National Transportation Safety Board, 2020).

BOX 1-1
Project Statement of Task

Pursuant to Section 554 of the FAA Reauthorization Act of 2018, the National Academies of Sciences, Engineering, and Medicine will conduct a consensus study to:

- Identify relevant drug and alcohol programs within U.S. Department of Transportation (DOT) and its modal administrations, and similar industries and sectors, beyond HIMS and FADAP;
- Review available assessments and evaluation information on the HIMS, FADAP, and any other identified drug and alcohol programs to identify:
  — Best policies and practices within existing programs; and
  — Best practices for prevention, early intervention, and return to work specifically around prescription medication abuse, with an emphasis on employee use of opioids; and
  — To the extent justified by the evidence, provide recommendations to the FAA and other modal administrations within the DOT on how to implement programs, or change existing programs, that seek to help transportation workers get treatment for drug and alcohol abuse and return to work.

The committee will deliver a report to FAA and the appropriate committees of Congress on the study, including findings, conclusions, and recommendations.

CONTEXT

Because of the high safety and security demands inherent in piloting, the FAA has instituted a multipronged approach to protect the public and the aviation workforce, recognizing that flying a commercial airliner engages all neurocognitive domains. A pilot operates a complex machine in an environment susceptible to rapid change affected by weather conditions, plane mechanics, geography, air traffic, time of day, and other human factors. Pilots must be prepared to rapidly respond cognitively and physically to altered circumstances in planes traveling at high speeds; thus any major impairment, whether associated with substance disorder or misuse, could jeopardize the lives of everyone onboard.[3] Flight attendants, too, must be prepared to respond quickly and effectively in high-pressure situations that can change abruptly.

Pilots must meet health standards. Commercial airline pilots must also have a first-class airman medical certificate.[4] The evaluations for these certificates are performed by aviation medical examiners. Part of this medical examination is a record of the pilot's behavioral health history, which includes any substance dependence or abuse as defined by the FAA.[5]

Key definitions and requirements for the first-class airman medical certificate include the following:

- For the FAA, "substance" includes alcohol, other sedatives and hypnotics, anxiolytics, opioids, central nervous system stimulants such as cocaine and amphetamines, and other psychoactive drugs.
- For the FAA, "substance dependence" means a condition in which a person is dependent on a substance, other than tobacco or ordinary xanthine-containing (e.g., caffeine) beverages, as evidenced by any one of the following:
  — increased tolerance;
  — manifestation of withdrawal symptoms;
  — impaired control of use; or
  — continued use despite damage to physical health or impairment of social, personal, or occupational functioning.
- The FAA also requires that pilots not have a record of substance abuse within the preceding two years. Flight attendants must pass random drug tests and function at expected levels.

If a pilot is experiencing problematic alcohol or other substance use, the FAA has measures in place to encourage them to seek the help they need. Pilots cannot be medically cleared to fly by the FAA if they have an alcohol use disorder, and they may face criminal charges if they report to work in a compromised state. Airlines are required to conduct random alcohol testing before flights, and very few pilots fail those tests (DOT, 2021).

It is important to note that, as discussed in detail in Chapter 2, the FAA definition of "dependence" is grounded in concerns about safety and functional impairments that are associated with use of certain substances,

---

[3]While there are numerous fatalities in general aviation, including recreational aviation, due to substance use-related impairment, major crashes of commercial airlines are extremely rare in the modern era of flight and there is no publicly available dataset on near misses.

[4]For more on this certificate, see https://www.ecfr.gov/current/title-14/chapter-I/subchapter-D/part-67/subpart-B/section-67.101

[5]For more on the mental health standards for airmen, see https://www.ecfr.gov/current/title-14/chapter-I/subchapter-D/part-67/subpart-B/section-67.107

even if substance use does not reach the levels that would meet the criteria for a diagnosis as defined by classification systems like the *Diagnostic and Statistical Manual, Fifth Edition.* For this reason, we follow conventions used by SAMHSA and refer to problematic use of drugs and alcohol as *substance misuse.*

HIMS and FADAP are designed to address substance misuse and substance use disorders among pilots and flight attendants, respectively. Training an airline pilot is an especially long, arduous, and costly process (BLS, 2022c), and therefore carriers have strong incentives to rehabilitate pilots who develop a substance use problem, as opposed to simply firing and replacing them. HIMS was established to assess the viability of an alcohol treatment and recovery program for pilots; it is a cooperative structure that includes airline representatives, pilot peer volunteers, health care professionals, and FAA medical specialists: see Box 1-2. It has evolved from a study into a professional monitoring program that seeks to coordinate the identification and treatment of pilots with substance use disorders as well as a return-to-work process for them, all under the FAA Special Issuance Regulations, and therefore carriers have strong incentives to rehabilitate pilots who develop a substance use problem, as opposed to simply firing and replacing them.

BOX 1-2
HIMS Overview

HIMS is described as "an occupational substance abuse treatment program, specific to pilots, that coordinates the identification, treatment, and return-to-work process for affected aviators." It is an industry-wide effort in which managers, pilots, healthcare professionals, and the FAA work together to preserve careers and enhance air safety. HIMS includes the involvement of company representatives, pilot peer volunteers, healthcare professionals, and FAA medical specialists. In some cases HIMS is also integrated into union and airline health and welfare supports such as Employee Assistance Programs (or EAPs). While the program borrows heavily from treatment principles developed in both clinical and industrial settings, it has specific elements that reflect the unique nature of the safety-sensitive airline transportation system. HIMS claims that similar-model programs not only exist in the United States but also have been successful in Canada and other countries around the world.

SOURCE: Data from https://himsprogram.com

BOX 1-3
FADAP Overview

FADAP was conceived by the Association of Flight Attendants-Communications Workers of America for the flight attendant profession. It began in September 2010 with funding from the FAA for all flight attendants regardless of employer or affiliation and regardless of status—active, furloughed, on leave. It is supported by flight attendant peers and managers from 25 carriers. Like HIMS, the identification and referral process is sometimes integrated within an airline's EAP program. The services it offers are described on its website as follows, addressed to potential program participants:

- 24/7 access to a flight attendant peer who understands and can talk with you about substance abuse—whether it is a concern about a flying partner's use or your own;
- referral to treatment programs that understand the culture of the flight attendant profession;
- post-treatment support services to help you sustain your recovery while balancing work and home life; and
- educational materials and conferences on substance abuse prevention, intervention, and treatment.

SOURCE: Data from https://www.fadap.org

The mission of FADAP as published on its website is "to support a culture of safety which will be able to assist flight attendants in meeting their personal and professional goals through substance-abuse awareness, combined with self and peer referrals for assistance, and the implementation of a flight-attendant-specific recovery support system"[6] (see Box 1-3).

STUDY APPROACH

The committee took note that HIMS and FADAP are prominent in the statement of task. Furthermore, the committee learned through its research, consultations with experts, and discussions with the study sponsor that HIMS is considered the gold standard among programs that address substance use disorders within the global transportation

---

[6]For more on FADAP, see https://www.fadap.org/

industry.[7] The committee also learned through its consultations that an impetus for the study was its potential to offer lessons from the HIMS and FADAP that could guide practice and policy for a range of transportation-related safety-sensitive occupations. Thus, the committee began by developing a complete understanding of the context within which the HIMS and FADAP operate and assessing the information available about the programs' operations and outcomes. It found, however, that evidence about the effectiveness of HIMS and FADAP is largely absent, and that the available information did not consistently support the conclusion that these programs should necessarily serve as models for other segments of the transportation industry. The committee decided to focus therefore on the HIMS and FADAP. Given the time available to conduct the study, in contrast with the kind of in-depth study of the programs and professional contexts of each mode that would be required to make recommendations about potential changes to practice and policy, the committee could not focus as much on other transportation industry programs.[8]

To further its understanding of HIMS and FADAP, the committee assembled information on the histories and the design of the programs, including their current structure and operating processes. The information gathered included available published reports on the programs, answers to the committee's questions about the programs from FAA officials, and discussions with parties that oversee and participate in the programs. Examination of the program context also included:

- attending annual meetings of the two programs;
- a public convening that included a human resources official from United Airlines to provide an example of how an EAP coordinates with HIMS and FADAP, as well as a small number of program participants and stakeholders; and
- responses to questions from program participants, primarily from FADAP.

The committee members met six times over a 12-month period to receive invited presentations in public meetings and to deliberate and apply their collective expertise in closed sessions. Subgroups of the committee met throughout this period on an as-needed basis to assess the information

---

[7]Information from a committee-hosted public workshop, available https://www. nationalacademies.org/event/11-01-2022/workshop-on-dealing-with-substance-use-disordersand-strengthening-well-being-in-commercial-aviation

[8]For a description of selected relevant programs in transportation, see Appendix A. The practices identified in this report are applicable, at least generally, to safety-sensitive transportation professions, but how to implement them depends on the professional context of each mode and would require in-depth study.

gathered and the implications for addressing the questions in the Statement of Task. The committee also commissioned papers from several outside experts to augment its own expertise. It further considered documentation of organizational structure and program details as provided by the FAA, HIMS, and FADAP leadership and by other government agencies. Information about programs of other transportation modes was gathered from relevant DOT agencies that responded to the committee's inquiries. Individuals who provided briefings and testimony to the committee and the topics covered, as well as the papers commissioned by the committee, are presented in Appendix B. Because a central feature of both FADAP and HIMS is the facilitation of clinical interventions for substance use disorder misuse, the committee reviewed literature, including research on substance-related problems among people employed in safety-sensitive occupations, on substance use disorders among flight attendants and pilots, and, as noted earlier, on evidence-based treatments. One commissioned paper focused on a clinical review of evidence on medication-assisted treatments[9] for substance use disorders, measuring the impairment effects of substance treatment that is medication-assisted, because the clinical practice of prescribing medication is subject to debate as it applies to the treatment of pilots and flight attendants (Kay & Belanger, 2022). The second commissioned paper undertook a quantitative analysis of the data received from FADAP (Nordberg, 2022). Because no source data were received from HIMS, the committee relied only on the very limited publicly reported information on pilots. The last paper is a qualitative analysis of responses from the "Call for Perspectives" and a series of focused follow-on interviews with 35 of the flight attendants and a single pilot (Wisdom, 2022).

Finally, the committee also received briefings from experts in the science of treating substance use disorders.[10] Some of those speakers emphasized special considerations that arise when treating people in safety-sensitive occupations. The purpose of these efforts was to support the committee members in putting the processes and interventions used by HIMS and FADAP into the context of modern evidence-based clinical practice for addressing any type of substance misuse and its application to safety-sensitive occupations. Because alcohol is the primary drug that is misused

---

[9]Medication-assisted treatment (MAT) is also known as medications for substance use disorders, generally, or more specifically as medications for alcohol use disorder (MAUD) and medications for opioid use disorder (MOUD). The committee used MAT for clarity and readability as it is commonly known in the field and used by HHS and FDA. However, the committee acknowledges that SAMHSA uses MOUD and MAUD and those terms will likely be more prevalent in the future.

[10]For more information, see the "Commissioned Papers" tab on the report webpage https://nap.nationalacademies.org/catalog/27025/substance-misuse-programs-in-commercial-aviation-safety-first

by pilots and flight attendants, the committee emphasized outcomes associated with alcohol misuse for alcohol use disorders.

Another source of information pursued by the committee was data from FADAP and HIMS. The committee reviewed publicly reported information from the two programs and analyzed program data that were made available to it. Publicly available reports provided a limited set of statistics on HIMS participants, such as treatment referral sources, substances misused, and rates of successful treatment and relapse. The committee requested access to the detailed program data to carry out the statistical analyses that are basic to evaluating any program, but it encountered multiple impediments to obtaining HIMS data for review and analysis. This included refusal by the FAA to share detailed HIMS data. In addition, the ALPA, which maintains the HIMS database through a contract with the FAA, refused to grant access to the data. In an effort to address concerns about data confidentiality and security, the committee proposed that ALPA conduct the committee's requested analysis on the de-identified data, but this proposal was denied. Finally, the committee's request to the FAA to compel HIMS to provide the relevant data was also denied, despite the contract stating that the data are owned by the U.S. government. Thus, after these repeated and varied efforts, the committee was unable to obtain source data regarding HIMS or have analyses conducted on its behalf by ALPA staff, and was, therefore, unable to review, analyze, and assess this program.[11] For a summary of communications regarding access to the HIMS database, see Appendix C.

As described above, the committee's work was constrained by a lack of access to complete data on pilots participating in HIMS. This is important for several reasons. First, lack of data made it difficult for the committee to interpret the limited publicly reported program results we were able to review. Without access to these data the committee cannot, for instance, resolve questions that arose during the study about the quality of HIMS

---

[11]During a Zoom meeting on April 27, 2022, with National Academies staff, the HIMS program manager offered to share queries and results from the HIMS database; follow-up attempts to agree on a data-sharing agreement that had specific confidentiality protections did not receive a response from HIMS. Following multiple requests, ALPA's HIMS Advisory Board denied the committee's request for data from the FAA-funded HIMS database on November 3, 2022, asserting the aforementioned contract with the FAA and concerns over confidentiality and data disclosure that might erode program integrity. A copy of the FAA/ALPA contract for HIMS was received by the committee on December 14, 2022. After review of the contract, the committee noted that the FAA owned the data, not ALPA, and indicated that access to the data would assist the National Academies in fulfilling the congressional mandate. During a follow-up meeting with National Academies staff on December 21, 2022, the FAA did not refute the National Academies' assertions about the FAA having full ownership of the HIMS data; nevertheless, the FAA noted that full access would not be provided. Rather, the FAA offered to make available aggregate data related to HIMS. Those aggregate data were never delivered.

data and data systems. Those questions were based on aggregate data reported by FAA and HIMS suggesting potential weaknesses in reporting or data quality or both. Second, the committee could not assess the ability of HIMS to effectively monitor and manage its operations, a concern that stemmed from claims about rates of relapse and statistics on referrals from annual medical evaluations reported by the FAA about HIMS. Finally, the committee was unable to fully assess the qualitative data it received from the "Call for Perspectives" in light of the quantitative data, as it could do to a limited extent with FADAP. Comparing qualitative and quantitative data is required, because qualitative reports from successful participants in a program are typically based on self-selected respondents and therefore may not offer reliable indications of a program's efficacy. In pursuing its charge, the committee sought to address a series of issues related to the ability of the FAA, HIMS, and FADAP to identify cases of substance use disorders, their approach to addressing those conditions, the degree to which the approach conforms with contemporary clinical science, and how the programs perform in promoting safety and returning pilots and flight attendants to work.

Identification of People in Need of Treatment

There are several ways that pilots and flight attendants are identified as having a problem in need of treatment. Those include failed random testing; self-referral; referral by family, friends and peers; events involving law enforcement (e.g., driving under the influence); referrals for suspicious behavior by Transportation Security Agency officers; and identification and referral by the employee's airline or union. The DOT and the FAA require random testing of people performing safety-sensitive functions, including flight attendants and pilots. The implementation of that testing program is left to airlines and unions, however. A key question is to what extent problematic substance misuse is identified through the detection and referral mechanisms associated with FADAP and HIMS. The committee was unable to completely answer this question due to lack of data, but, as an example, it could ascertain from the available information that 0.5 percent of pilots are referred by aviation medical examiners during mandated annual screenings. Given an estimated prevalence rate of 15.4 percent (SAMHSA, 2021), a referral rate of 0.5 percent implies a case detection rate of less than one half of one percent. As mentioned previously, this observation raises questions such as the effectiveness of screening procedures and the quality of data and data reporting.

The Role of FADAP and HIMS in the
Ecology of Aviation Safety and Healthcare

HIMS and FADAP are only two parts of a complex array of mechanisms for addressing substance use disorders in aviation. Moreover, there are vast differences between the two programs, with each having distinct structures and operating procedures and carrying very different employment and cost consequences for their participants. Other key institutions include EAPs run by unions and airlines, standard health insurance that covers and pays for treatment, mutual support groups such as Alcoholics Anonymous and SMART Recovery, and private financial resources. HIMS facilitates treatment for about 1.4 percent of all pilots (Skaggs & Norris, 2021),[12] even though their own estimates on the prevalence rate for substance use disorders is 8–12 percent.[13] That means HIMS only accounts for a small fraction of pilots with substance use disorders. The data produced by FADAP highlight the fact that some of the largest carriers do not appear to participate in the FADAP (see Chapter 2). These observations mean that the FAA, the unions, and the HIMS and FADAP likely have limited visibility into both the degree to which substance misuse problems are identified and the treatment approaches taken, and outcomes realized for the total pilot and flight attendant population. Neither the programs nor the committee were positioned to offer insights into these issues due to the incomplete data of uncertain quality.

Heavy Reliance on Inpatient and Residential Treatment Modalities

Both HIMS and FADAP rely heavily on treatment in inpatient and residential settings. In addition to this reliance, the FAA and HIMS find MATs unacceptable for ongoing treatment of substance misuse. The committee focused on understanding the degree to which the clinical content of HIMS and FADAP aligns with modern evidence-based treatment for substance use problems. In contemporary evidence-based practice for the treatment of some substance use disorders, MAT is a first-line intervention (e.g., opioid use disorder and alcohol use disorder), and it is even considered advantageous in avoiding relapse and, in the case of opioids, in preventing overdose with appropriate medication selection and monitoring (U.S. Food and Drug Administration [FDA], n.d.). Where departures from evidence-based approaches exist, the committee sought to understand the extent to which those departures may be grounded in and justified by the unique circumstances of safety-sensitive occupations.

---

[12]Based on the percentage of active pilots that have a substance use disorder-related special issuance in 2018. Another 0.37 percent of pilots were monitored for misuse.

[13]Information from the 2023 HIMS, available at https://himsprogram.com/

HIMS and FADAP Make Strong Assertions for Their Successes

Strong assertions of success include HIMS noting that the model has been adopted by more than 40 airlines across the United States, as well as in Canada and eight other countries around the world. HIMS also asserts a return of nine dollars for every program dollar of spending and an "85 percent long-term abstinence rate."[14] Opportunity to examine the evidence supporting such statements is fundamental for determining the extent of HIMS' success and whether the model should be extended elsewhere in the transportation sector, as was asked of this National Academies committee. Thus, the committee sought to confirm that these assertions are grounded in evidence, but the combination of incomplete data and questions about data quality and departures from evidence in the literature precluded the committee from being able to fully form conclusions related to this part of its charge.

ORGANIZATION OF THE REPORT

Following this introduction, Chapter 2 provides the history and descriptions of HIMS and FADAP. Chapter 3 covers the scientific evidence on practices in treatment programs for substance use disorders, and Chapter 4 reviews the key components in evaluating such programs. Chapter 5 turns to the committee's analysis of the evidence about HIMS and FADAP, and Chapter 6 presents the committee's conclusions and recommendations.

There are several appendixes to this report. Appendix A documents the information collected on other substance use disorder programs in transportation. Appendix B details the various avenues for data gathering to help assist the committee in its deliberations. Appendix C outlines the timing of the committee's requests for access to data through various programs and offices. Appendix D provides brief biographies of the committee members. Finally, Appendix E notes the unavoidable conflict of interest in the committee membership.

---

[14] Ibid.

2

Brief Descriptions of the Human Intervention and Motivational Study and the Flight Attendant Drug and Alcohol Program

This chapter provides a brief description of two prominent drug and alcohol programs overseen by the Federal Aviation Administration (FAA). These programs, the Human Intervention and Motivational Study (HIMS) and the Flight Attendant Drug and Alcohol Program (FADAP), support pilots and flight attendants, respectively, who misuse substances and who have substance use disorders. This chapter describes both programs' structures. An analysis of program engagement, outcomes, and effectiveness will be provided in Chapter 5. The discussion starts with the applicable regulatory principles governing the alcohol and substance use programs in aviation, followed by a general description of each program that includes the treatment service delivery process—identification, referral, treatment provider selection and placement, and continuing care/recovery support services; return-to-duty procedure; program monitoring; and workplace outcomes measurement.

**REGULATORY CONTEXT:
SUBSTANCE MISUSE PROGRAMS IN THE AVIATION SECTOR**

The regulatory principles that govern substance use programs in the aviation industry come from the FAA and the Department of Health and Human Services (HHS). 14 CFR § 120 outlines FAA policies designed to prevent accidents and injuries resulting from the misuse of drugs or alcohol by employees in aviation with safety-sensitive functions.[1] These

---

[1] https://www.ecfr.gov/current/title-14/chapter-I/subchapter-G/part-120

23

regulations state which employees must be tested, which substances they must be tested for, and when these tests should occur. Administrative procedures for these tests are also described, as are the consequences for employees that fail a test.

While the general FAA rules and definitions apply to many aviation employees, pilots have separate rules and definitions for problematic substance use. Becoming a commercial carrier pilot (also called an Airline Transport Pilot) for a major U.S. airline usually requires possessing a first-class airman[2] medical certificate; therefore, it is those highest standards that are the focus of the committee's work.[3] This medical certification includes a record of the pilot's behavioral health history, including substance dependence or abuse (14 Code of Federal Regulations [CFR] § 67.107).[4] If there is a history of substance dependence, there must be established clinical evidence of recovery, defined as complete abstinence from the substance for not less than the preceding two years (14 CFR § 67.107).[5] It should be noted that the *Diagnostic and Statistical Manual of Mental Disorders, Fifth Edition* (DSM-5) does not define recovery from substance use disorders, nor is there a consensus on what clinically constitutes recovery and how to measure it.

The programs are also informed by regulations related to the specific credentials a professional must possess to be qualified to assess and determine the return-to-duty process for safety-sensitive transportation employees. For example, U.S. Department of Transportation (DOT) Rule 49 CFR § 40.281(o) outlines the credentials, basic knowledge, qualification training, and continuing education needed to become a Substance Abuse Professional (SAP) for the DOT.[6,7] Additionally, given the confidential nature of pilots' and flight attendants' participation in these programs, 42 CFR § 2.32, within the Substance Abuse and Mental Health Services Administration (SAMHSA) at HHS imposes restrictions on the disclosure and use of patient records for substance use disorder patients, which are maintained as part of any federally assisted program and establishes a

---

[2] "Airman" is an FAA term and refers to pilots of all genders.

[3] For a summary of the different medical standards by pilot class, see https://www.faa.gov/ame_guide/standards

[4] https://www.ecfr.gov/current/title-14/chapter-I/subchapter-D/part-67/subpart-B/section-67.107

[5] After a prepublication version of the report was provided to the FAA, this section was edited to clarify abstinence duration.

[6] The credential of a SAP was created by the DOT to clarify who is qualified to assess their employees. It is a credential that providers have to obtain if they want to perform evaluations on transportation employees.

[7] https://www.transportation.gov/odapc/part40/40-281

criminal penalty for violation of these restrictions.[8] These regulations form a foundation that the HIMS and FADAP are able to build on.[9]

HIMS

Definitions and Sources of Information

According to the FAA (2023a), there are approximately 167,000 commercial airline pilots flying for major carriers (e.g., United, American, Delta, Southwest), small carriers (e.g. Frontier, JetBlue, Spirit), regional airlines (e.g., Republic, CommuteAir, Envoy) and cargo carriers (e.g., FedEx, UPS, Atlas Air, Kalitta). In addition to the licensing and certifications necessary to fly aircraft, pilots are required to hold medical certification. Specifically, pilots flying for the aforementioned airlines are required to hold first class medical certification as defined by 14 CFR § 67. Section 67.107 addresses mental health, with 14 CFR § 67.107(a)(4) specifying *substance dependence* as a disqualifying condition:

> (4) Substance dependence, except where there is established clinical evidence, satisfactory to the Federal Air Surgeon, of recovery, including sustained total abstinence from the substance(s) for not less than the preceding 2 years. As summarized in this section -
> (i) "Substance" includes: Alcohol; other sedatives and hypnotics; anxiolytics; opioids; central nervous system stimulants such as cocaine, amphetamines, and similarly acting sympathomimetics; hallucinogens; phencyclidine or similarly acting arylcyclohexylamines; cannabis; inhalants; and other psychoactive drugs and chemicals; and
> (ii) "Substance dependence" means a condition in which a person is dependent on a substance, other than tobacco or ordinary xanthine-containing (e.g., caffeine) beverages, as evidenced by one or more of the following -
> (A) Increased tolerance;
> (B) Manifestation of withdrawal symptoms;
> (C) Impaired control of use; or
> (D) Continued use despite damage to physical health or impairment of social, personal, or occupational functioning.

14 CFR § 67.107(b) further defines *substance abuse* as a disqualification but with the proviso that the pilot can resume duties if free of abuse for the preceding two years:

---

[8]https://www.ecfr.gov/current/title-42/chapter-I/subchapter-A/part-2

[9]The committee acknowledges that potential changes could be coming to the regulations: https://www.hhs.gov/hipaa/for-professionals/regulatory-initiatives/hipaa-part-2/index.html

(b) No substance abuse within the preceding 2 years defined as:
  (1) Use of a substance in a situation in which that use was physically hazardous, if there has been at any other time an instance of the use of a substance also in a situation in which that use was physically hazardous;
  (2) A verified positive drug test result, an alcohol test result of 0.04 or greater alcohol concentration, or a refusal to submit to a drug or alcohol test required by the U.S. Department of Transportation or an agency of the U.S. Department of Transportation; or
  (3) Misuse of a substance that the Federal Air Surgeon, based on case history and appropriate, qualified medical judgment relating to the substance involved, finds -
    (i) Makes the person unable to safely perform the duties or exercise the privileges of the airman certificate applied for or held; or
    (ii) May reasonably be expected, for the maximum duration of the airman medical certificate applied for or held, to make the person unable to perform those duties or exercise those privileges.

The regulatory definitions of substance dependence and abuse differ from the current Text Revision of DSM-5 (DSM-5-TR; see American Psychiatric Association, 2022) while still capturing key elements of substance misuse. The DSM-5 criteria for a diagnosable substance use disorder require at least two of the following symptoms in a given year:

- using more of a substance than planned, or using a substance for a longer interval than desired;
- inability to cut down despite desire to do so;
- spending substantial amount of the day obtaining, using, or recovering from substance use;
- cravings or intense urges to use;
- repeated usage that causes or contributes to an inability to meet important social or professional obligations;
- persistent usage despite user's knowledge that it is causing frequent problems at work, school, or home;
- giving up or cutting back on important social, professional, or leisure activities because of use;
- usage in physically hazardous situations, or usage causing physical or mental harm;
- persistent use despite the user's awareness that the substance is causing or at least worsening a physical or mental problem;
- tolerance (needing to use increasing amounts of a substance to obtain its desired effects); and
- withdrawal (a characteristic group of physical effects or symptoms that emerge as the amount of substance in the body decreases).

The FAA's regulatory definitions of substance abuse and dependence are notably more restrictive than the accepted clinical guidance. Moreover, the FAA considers substance abuse within the last two years or, substance dependence regardless of timeframe, as grounds for disqualification from medical certification (14 CFR § 67.107).[10] Additionally, the regulatory environment requires strict enforcement by the FAA; as a result, identification of a substance use disorder places the pilot's job and livelihood at risk. This unique environment for pilots stands in sharp contrast to other occupations, where identification and treatment of substance use disorders is of lower risk to employability. The environment leads to considerable reticence to disclose one's own struggles or those of a fellow pilot. Nevertheless, pilots face challenges including easy access to alcohol, especially on layovers, difficult travel schedules, isolation, and high stress levels, particularly when away from support networks.

The following sections outline the history and organization of HIMS. Sources of information include the HIMS website,[11] written responses to inquiries from the HIMS Program Manager, HIMS Overview slides presented at conferences, and content from the HIMS Basic Seminar (Snyder, 2022).

Special Issuance Authorization

With the introduction of HIMS in 1974, a mechanism was developed for identifying and treating substance use disorders, along with a system for monitoring and returning to duty. Although the conditions of substance dependence and abuse are still considered disqualifying, 14 CFR § 67.401 provides for Authorization for Special Issuance of a Medical Certificate at the discretion of the Federal Air Surgeon. This authorization can be issued to pilots who demonstrate that they can perform their duties without endangering public safety. The creation of HIMS allowed for pilots diagnosed with substance abuse and dependence to pursue treatment and to eventually make a return to the flightdeck, supplanting prior practice of pilots being dismissed.

Because the medical certification of pilots is key to maintaining the safety of aircraft, passengers, and employees, HIMS is primarily framed as a safety program designed to ensure that the adverse effects of a pilot's substance misuse do not pose an undue risk (Snyder, 2022). For pilots, however, it represents a way to maintain medical certification and employment and return to flight duties. HIMS standards currently apply across all three classes of medical certification for pilots.

---

[10]After a prepublication version of the report was provided to the FAA, this section was edited to accurately reflect the information found in the CFR.

[11]https://himsprogram.com

Program Design and Structure

There is no central administration of HIMS beyond the FAA-funded core elements of educational programming (aimed primarily for airlines and medical professionals), maintaining a database of participants, and serving as an overall substance misuse information hub, although there are commonalities in HIMS structure across airlines designed to meet the requirements of the FAA's special issuance process. Commonalities include the referral-to-treatment, monitoring, and return-to-duty processes. The specific structure of each program differs according to each airline's arrangements with its pilots, often made through collective bargaining agreements (Snyder, 2022). As such, the various pilot unions and companies have considerable autonomy in how they carry out the expectations of the program.

The cornerstone structure of the typical HIMS team within an airline comprises the HIMS-trained aviation medical examiner (HIMS AME), the company, the pilot's union, and mental health professionals. While the pilots' unions contribute to the structure of HIMS at a given airline, the company often maintains the managerial functions and assumes financial responsibility for the treatment (through their provided insurance) and for monitoring components of the program. Some airlines use their Employee Assistance Program (EAP) in the initial referral/identification process as well as in the ongoing monitoring phase of the program. However, because of the variability among carriers and pilot unions, financial support for the pilot in treatment varies greatly. Regardless of the structure within and between airlines, the HIMS process is ultimately guided by the HIMS AME or medical sponsor and on the advisement of the mental health professionals including the HIMS-trained psychiatrist and neuropsychologist (P&P). See Figures 2-1 and 2-2 for the operating model and oversight structure of HIMS.

Identification and Referral to the Program

Pilots can enter HIMS in a variety of ways. Initial identification of whether a pilot meets the regulatory definition of substance abuse or dependence can be initiated by FAA request following a report of a substance-related arrest, substance-related medical event, or other information that may suggest a substance-related issue (Snyder, 2022). Pilots can also enter the program through a variety of other pathways, including self-referral, referral by the airline/supervisor, or on the recommendation of their AME. Regardless of the referral mechanism, entering the program may depend on the identification of a substance use issue that meets the regulatory definitions of abuse or dependence. Pilots may also be referred to the program following a positive test result during random DOT testing, which accounts

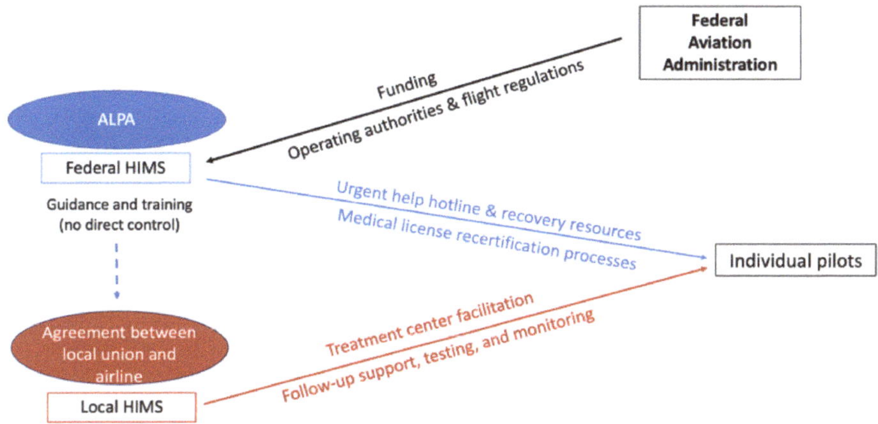

FIGURE 2-1 Governance operating model for HIMS.
SOURCE: Data from https://himsprogram.com/ and responses to the committee questionnaire to HIMS.

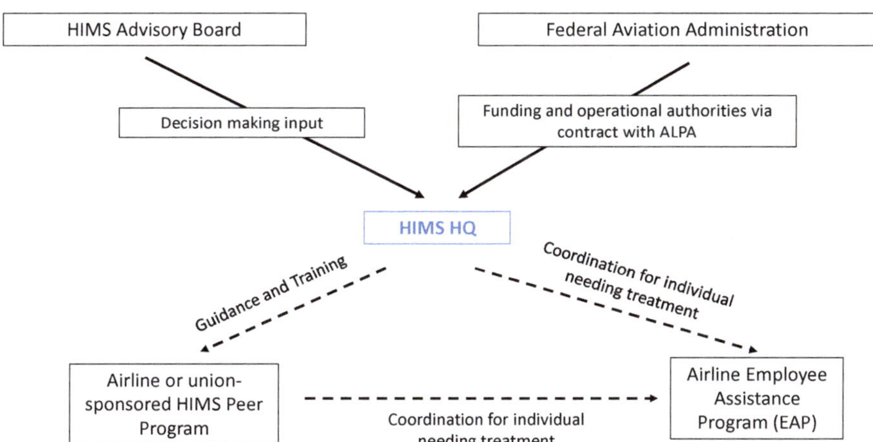

FIGURE 2-2 HIMS oversight structure.
SOURCE: Data from https://himsprogram.com/ and responses to the committee questionnaire to HIMS.

for approximately eight percent of all pilots entering the program. Entry into the program can also be facilitated by a family member or coworker.

Regardless of the mechanism of referral, in many instances a formal assessment by a SAP is conducted. These initial evaluations are performed by professionals in disciplines knowledgeable in the assessment and treatment of substance use disorders such as psychiatry, psychology, and social work or by other licensed masters-level clinicians holding the DOT required qualifications to become a SAP. In addition to the ability to make a clinical diagnosis, the clinician must be trained in and be familiar with the FAA's regulatory standards and definitions.

Program Introduction and Awareness

Program awareness can vary from airline to airline. All pilots are free to attend HIMS seminars, which are multiday events bringing together pilots, AMEs, and other program stakeholders to train and discuss their experiences. In addition, airline pilots are introduced to HIMS through a 20–60-minute training segment on HIMS during initial-hire and annual trainings. HIMS also distributes literature, including employee manuals, publications to unions, and brochures, as well as merchandise.

Treatment Modalities and Monitoring

Neither HIMS nor the FAA require admission to any specific treatment facility. Selection of treatment centers is at the discretion of the airline or union that manages a HIMS. Initial treatment types and settings vary. First class pilots most commonly enter treatment at the residential level and length of stay is based on a 28-day model; detox is completed if needed. Following this initial treatment episode, all classes of pilots most commonly transition into the aftercare level of treatment, continuing with group therapy once per week and periodic contact with a psychiatric provider and individual therapist (Snyder, 2022).

Aftercare and monitoring are considered essential components for maintaining sobriety. The HIMS aftercare component typically coincides with the initiation of the aftercare level of treatment. In addition to the formal treatment noted above, it commonly includes meetings with peer pilot monitors, company representatives, and EAP staff, as well as engagement in mutual help programs such as 12-step programs, most commonly Alcoholics Anonymous (AA). Birds of a Feather, available to pilots and flightdeck crew members across the world, is an AA-based mutual support group pilots are encouraged to participate in.[12]

---

[12]For more information on Birds of a Feather, see www.BOAF.org

The monitoring phase begins following the initial treatment phase, coinciding with HIMS aftercare, and continues after the special-issuance authorization. Monitoring follows a step-down process with monitoring requirements gradually reduced over the course of several years (Snyder, 2022). However, in a small number of cases, monitoring may continue for the duration of a pilot's career. Monitoring includes both regular and random drug and alcohol testing[13] as well as ongoing contact with the company representatives/EAP, peer monitors, psychiatric providers, and the HIMS aeromedical examiner. It also includes attendance at mutual support groups. Open communication among the monitoring entities is encouraged and, in some companies, is formally convened.

Throughout treatment and monitoring, peer and company monitors, as well as treatment providers, are responsible for generating monthly reports, which are included in the pilot's submission package for Special Issuance and follow-up monitoring. This monitoring model is intended to actively address the risk of relapse.

Evaluation for Fitness for Duty

The pilot's HIMS team plays an essential role in determining the pilot's quality of recovery and subsequent readiness for evaluation for fitness to return to flight duties. Continuing cognitive impairment related to substance misuse and poor recovery is a common reason for prohibiting a pilot from proceeding to the evaluation for fitness for duty. Premature referral for evaluation can cause a subsequent delay, a return to further treatment, and need to repeat all or part of the neurocognitive assessment. Once a determination has been made to proceed with evaluation, the pilot is referred to a P&P for assessment of psychiatric and neurocognitive status. Each evaluator is provided with complete records, including the pilot's full FAA medical record and all treatment and monitoring records.

As HIMS has evolved, the neurocognitive testing process has evolved. The neuropsychological assessment utilizes a battery of standard and commonly used measures that have been validated for aeromedically significant cognitive functions such as deductive reasoning, working memory and attention, processing speed and efficiency, verbal and visual memory, and general intellectual functioning. Aspects of these cognitive abilities are also considered to be vulnerable to chronic substance misuse.

Following completion of these assessments, the pilot is either referred for further treatment or cognitive rehabilitation activities or recommended for consideration for special issuance certification. If recommended for further consideration, the pilot is medically evaluated by the HIMS aeromedical

---

[13]Including remote monitoring systems such as Soberlink.

examiner, and the final submission package is assembled. That package includes all documentation including treatment records, monitoring reports, and P&P reports. The medical sponsor is responsible for assembling the records and generating a comprehensive summary for submission to the FAA for final determination of eligibility for special issuance authorization.

Special Issuance

Authorization for a special issuance is contingent on the pilot following certain requirements. In the near term, continued monitoring is required, including random drug and alcohol testing, continued individual and/or group therapy, meetings with peer monitors, follow-up with the HIMS aeromedical examiner/sponsor and HIMS psychiatrist, and continued engagement in a peer support/12-step program. A HIMS step-down process was approved in 2020 that gradually reduces monitoring requirements over a minimum of seven years.

HIMS Summary

HIMS is a safety-oriented program designed to facilitate the identification, treatment, monitoring, and return-to-duty of pilots with substance abuse and dependence as defined by 14 CFR § 67. While the broad goals and FAA special issuance authorization standards are consistent, the program's implementation can vary between carriers. Additionally, the treatment of substance use disorder can constitute significant expense of time and money. While mutual help groups such as AA are free and have no attendance requirements, more time spent in meetings is related to higher rates of abstinence (Kaskutas, 2009). Residential inpatient treatment cost an average of $42,500. (French et al., 2008). Oftentimes only pilots at major carriers with strong unions who support HIMS will be provided with necessary financial support. Smaller carriers with more limited budgets may leave pilots with much less financial support for treatment and more limited leave from work. A lack of financial support can be a significant barrier to entering treatment, especially among pilots at smaller and regional carriers.[14] Reliance on temporary disability coverage, sick leave, or a total lack of support may impact the pilot's decision to engage in treatment and even treatment effectiveness.

Another barrier to entering HIMS (and, subsequently, treatment) is the unique medical certification requirements that pilots must meet to exercise

---

[14]Information from a committee-hosted public workshop, available https://www.nationalacademies.org/event/11-01-2022/workshop-on-dealing-with-substance-use-disordersand-strengthening-well-being-in-commercial-aviation

pilot privileges. Identification of a disqualifying condition places the pilot's medical certificate and, in turn, the pilot's career and livelihood at risk. As a result, pilots may be disincentivized to reveal that they are affected by substance use, even if HIMS may otherwise help them pursue treatment.

Another component worthy of further study is the small number of residential treatment facilities treating pilots who will eventually apply for special issuance medical certification. The HIMS Program Manager noted that there are approximately a dozen treatment facilities across the United States approved to treat HIMS participants, though there are more than 11,000 substance use disorder treatment facilities in the United States (Cantor et al., 2022).

HIMS further notes that many facilities are unwilling to engage with airline HIMS teams during and after treatment to generate the documentation necessary for FAA review as part of the final determination process. This makes it difficult to expand the "roster" of treatment facilities to which HIMS can refer their pilots. It is unclear how much of a barrier the small number of treatment facilities poses or how a treatment program gets approved by airlines.

Finally, the HIMS Advisory Board approved the development of a confidential database with the stated goal of identifying areas for improvement in HIMS.[15] The database and data collection are funded by the FAA as a part of the HIMS contract with the Air Line Pilots Association, International.[16] While all data are de-identified, the database is for internal use only and reviewed annually by three individuals at the FAA and HIMS.[17] Searchable fields in the HIMS database include age cohort, size of airline, method of entering program, primary substance, dual diagnosis, number of relapses, and family history.[18]

FADAP

Flight attendants are responsible for ensuring cabin safety. They conduct safety checks before the flight and ensure effective communication of safety procedures with customers, as well as operate safety devices, as needed, in times of emergency. In addition to commonly known risk factors for developing substance use disorders, flight attendants also face challenges unique to their work environment that increase susceptibility to relapse and that can be triggering during recovery. Like pilots, flight attendants also face challenges including easy access to alcohol, difficult travel schedules,

---

[15]HIMS staff response to the committee-issued questionnaire, August 2022.
[16]Ibid.
[17]Ibid.
[18]Ibid.

isolation, and high stress levels, particularly when dealing with difficult customers and being away from personal supports. It is critical, therefore, that impairment among flight attendants be addressed in a timely and appropriate manner so that safety-sensitive duties are not compromised.

FADAP's stated mission advances a culture of safety among flight attendants by addressing impairment through awareness of substance misuse and by supporting their personal and professional goals by allowing self or peer referrals to seek treatment (FADAP, n.d.). Hence, the program may be viewed as having two distinct components: (1) an educational component and (2) a treatment-referral and recovery-support component.

According to FADAP staff,

> early surveys conducted of flight attendants in 2012 and 2013 showed that approximately 10 to 12 percent of flight attendants are engaged in misuse/abuse behaviors around alcohol, drugs, and medications. Within all DOT safety-sensitive groups for aviation, flight attendants ranked either first or second for DOT drug test violations across various testing reasons (pre-employment, random, for cause/suspicion, post-accident, follow-up testing) compared to all other aviation safety-sensitive work groups.[19]

The following subsections synthesize and present information about FADAP operations made available to this study committee along with information from the FADAP website.

General Program Description

FADAP is a substance misuse prevention and assistance referral program available and accessible to all flight attendants regardless of their employment status (furloughed, active, on leave) and airline affiliation. The program provides referral to treatment and peer mentorship to flight attendants seeking or undergoing treatment and those in recovery from substance use disorders. Mentoring peers are fellow flight attendants, many having gone through treatment themselves, and they are trained by FADAP's central office. FADAP also engages in primary prevention of substance misuse by making available educational materials, videos, and self-assessment screening tools, as well as by conducting educational seminars to key airline stakeholders on early identification and intervention for substance use disorders. The program is recognized as an approved educational provider by the Labor Assistance Professional Association, Employee Assistance Professional Association, National Association of Alcohol and Drug Counselors, and the Maryland Board of Social Work Examiners.

---

[19]FADAP staff response to the committee-issued questionnaire, August 2022.

Established in September 2010,[20] "FADAP was endorsed by flight attendant peers and managers from 25 carriers during a March 2009 'Return to the Cabin' Summit" (FADAP, n.d.).

Program funding for FADAP is provided by the FAA. FAA contracts with the Association of Flight Attendants (AFA-CWA), a union representing about 50,000 flight attendants at 19 airlines, for administrative oversight of the program.[21] The central FADAP staff comprises a manager, coordinator, and administrator, who are primarily responsible for program oversight, including the development and implementation of educational activities to increase substance misuse awareness among flight attendants and their families.[22] The staff performs the following tasks:

- develops an outreach plan for educating and recruiting flight attendant volunteers as peers or workplace-based recovery mentors;
- develops educational materials and conducts educational seminars, peer training, annual conferences, and other, similar activities;
- maintains a FADAP database and website, used as the key informational resource for program awareness among flight attendants and their families;
- identifies and maintains a list of approved treatment providers based on input from various sectors, FADAP staff site visits and evaluations of staffing credentials, and facility accreditations (FADAP staff provides a minimum half-day training for facility staff on FADAP, flight attendant culture, occupational demands, stressors, and required communication and paperwork); and
- submits progress reports and meets with the advisory board, at least once a year.

The FADAP Advisory Board monitors the program's implementation, recommends changes in program operations as needed, and reviews program outcomes. It is composed of flight attendants, flight attendant managers, the FAA, and experts in the field of substance use disorders. The board approves the FADAP outreach plan, educational materials, and program activities.[23] See Figure 2-3 for the FADAP governance operating model.

The other key FADAP component is to facilitate access to substance use treatment through peer support. Each FADAP is sponsored by an airline

---

[20]The AFA-CWA did have an expanded EAP for flight attendants before FADAP (Feuer, 1987), but it is unclear what elements (if any) from the old system were maintained after the 2010 launch.

[21]FADAP staff response to the committee-issued questionnaire, August 2022.

[22]Ibid.

[23]Ibid.

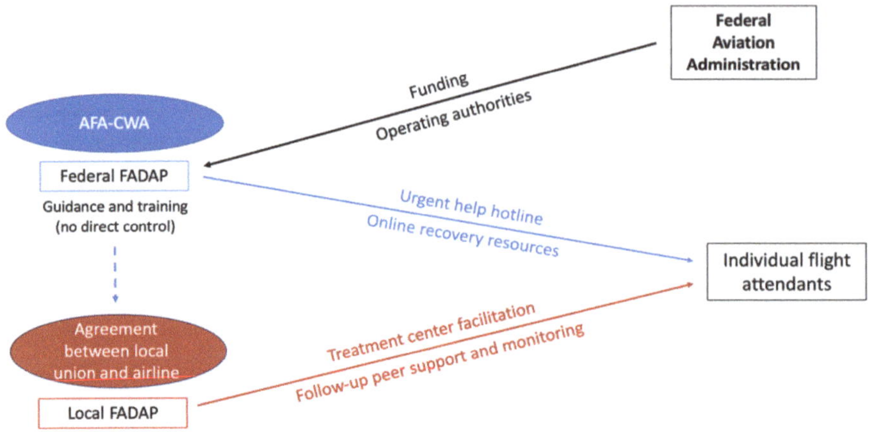

FIGURE 2-3 FADAP governance operating model.
SOURCE: Data from https://www.fadap.org/more-about-fadap and responses to the committee questionnaire to FADAP.

and its associated flight attendant union. While peer training is conducted by FADAP staff, the sponsoring airline or union has direct oversight of their own FADAP peer program. While there is no formal written agreement between the EAP and FADAP, they collaborate and, whenever possible, they comanage flight attendants referred for short-term substance use treatment.

Airlines are not mandated by the FAA to establish a FADAP peer program, nor are they obligated to support the cost of FADAP operations.[24] However, airline management may choose to extend support however they deem appropriate, such as coordinating travel for peers to attend FADAP training, paying for expenses associated with attending the program's seminars and conferences, allowing peers time off to attend its educational seminars, or offering FADAP training to flight attendant leaders and supervisors.

FADAP administrators believe its peer support system is a model for motivating flight attendants, particularly those who have no reported rule violation, to seek treatment without fear of disclosing their condition to their employer or the FAA.[25] Confidentiality is observed both for the flight attendant seeking treatment as well as for the referring agent (e.g., flight attendant colleague, manager or supervisor, pilot). This allows voluntary removal from performing safety-sensitive duties while impaired

---

[24]Ibid.
[25]Ibid.

(in which case the flight crew may call FADAP to "save a peer") or while undergoing treatment, and hence preserves the opportunity for flight attendants to keep their job and return safely to duty.

Figure 2-4 depicts the relationships among the various agencies and organizations involved in administering the FADAP.

Treatment Service Delivery Process

FADAP services are available and accessible to all flight attendants. They may either call the FADAP central helpline or contact, in person or by phone, the FADAP peer program at their airline. Twenty-four airlines have an established FADAP peer program. They vary in size, maturity, and visibility in the flight attendants' work environment. Some are fully assimilated into labor and management communications, training programs, and partnership activities.

Peers are flight attendant volunteers who made a commitment to participate in the FADAP case management process. They are appointed by the peer program sponsor (i.e., the union or airline management). Peers undergo a one-day training given by FADAP staff on topics including:

- nature and models of addiction;
- successful interventions, which motivate the flight attendant to seek treatment;

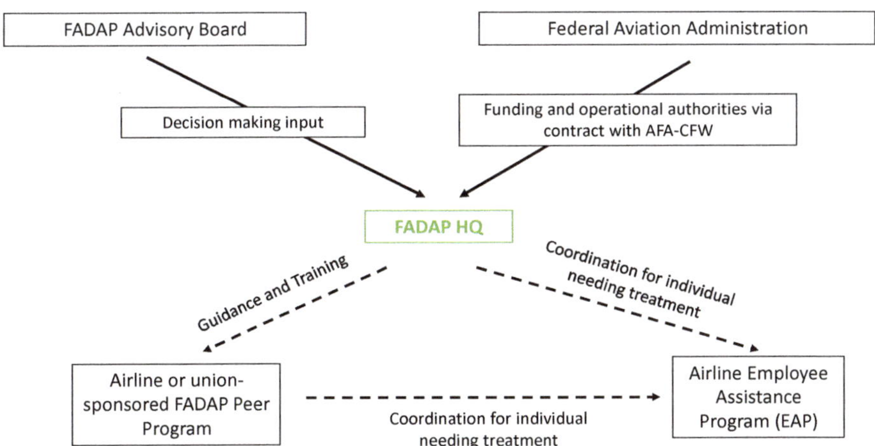

FIGURE 2-4 FADAP oversight structure.
SOURCE: Data from https://www.fadap.org/more-about-fadap and responses to the committee questionnaire to FADAP.

- types of substance use treatments, best treatment practices for flight attendants, the treatment continuum;
- safely moving the flight attendant into treatment;
- FADAP peer case manager checklist;
- re-occurrence (relapse) prevention;
- FADAP resources;
- what one needs to know to function as a peer; and
- peer self-care.

Incoming peers are "shadowed" by a more senior peer for several months and provided access to periodic virtual continuing education training, virtual FADAP treatment site-visits, and 2.5 days of education during the FADAP conference. A certification track for peers is also offered to advance their education and training.[26]

Identification and Referral

While there are no mandatory requirements for flight attendants to report substance use problems or substance-related convictions to the FAA or airline, there are several pathways for referring or identifying flight attendants to participate in FADAP (see Figure 2-5). Flight attendants may self-identify, or referrals may be received from colleagues, family members, flight attendant unions, EAPs, supervisors/managers, or others such as flight attendants involved in accident investigations, a failed drug test administered by the DOT, or disciplinary action due to substance misuse.

Screening and Assessment

When a flight attendant is referred to FADAP, the program conducts outreach through a peer, who later serves as the point of contact for the initiation of an intervention.[27] The peer conducts the initial screening to determine whether the flight attendant is misusing a substance and to determine the extent, seriousness, and urgency of any work-related issue. The peer motivates the flight attendant to seek treatment, and when a flight attendant agrees to go, the flight attendant selects a treatment program from a list of FADAP-approved treatment providers for admission to care.

The treatment intake process generally includes evaluation for primary mental health diagnoses and personality disorders. According to the FADAP *2021 Annual Report,*

---

[26]Ibid.
[27]Ibid.

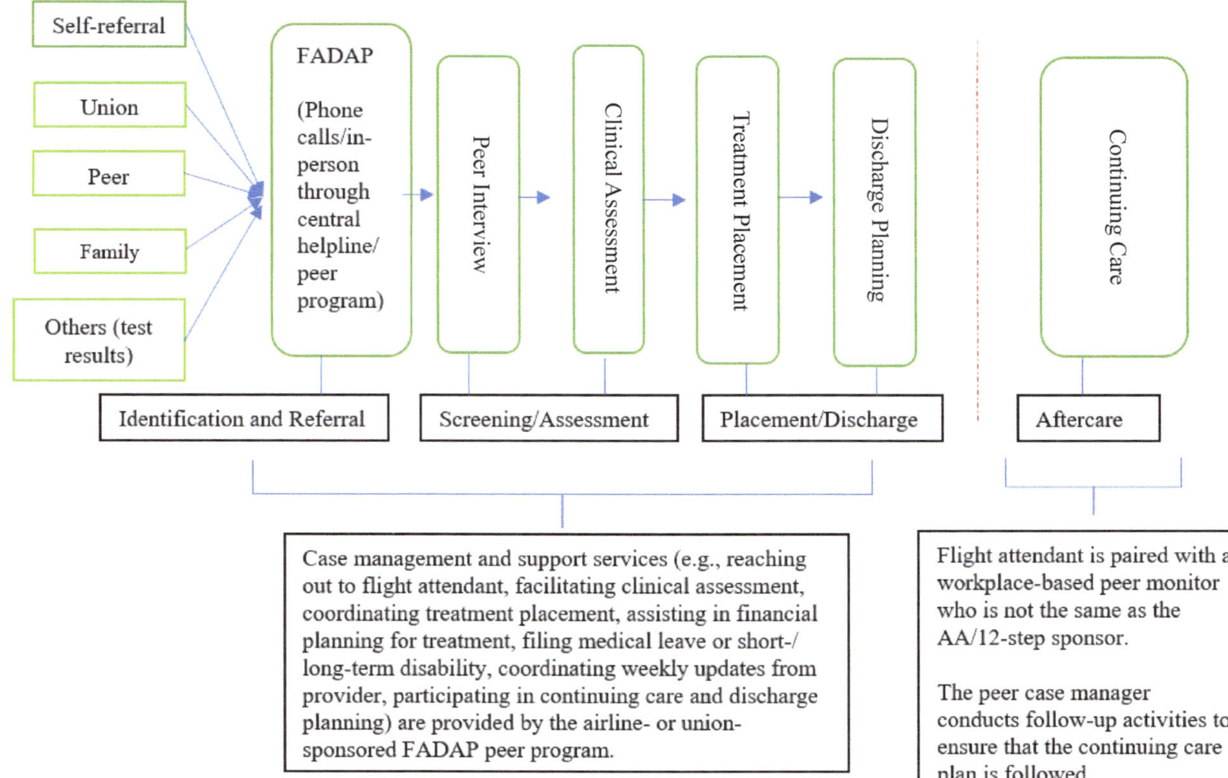

FIGURE 2-5 Treatment service delivery process through FADAP.
SOURCE: Data from https://www.fadap.org/more-about-fadap and responses to the committee questionnaire to FADAP.

over the past two years, 37 percent of Flight Attendants were diagnosed with anxiety and related disorders, 45 percent with depressive disorders, 4 percent with bipolar and related disorders, and 8 percent with other mental health disorders or other disorders. Diagnosis is defined using the DSM-5 criteria.[28]

In response to a committee questionnaire received from FADAP staff, beginning in 2021 the Advisory Board approved the expansion of FADAP's focus to include mental health messaging. As of June 2022, all FADAP peers had completed training in a course focused on mental health first aid in the workplace. While tobacco use is known to be widely prevalent among persons with mental health disorders and increases the risk of relapse to other substance use, it has not been formally included in the FADAP assessment process. However, FADAP staff reported that they had referred flight attendants for smoking cessation.

Treatment Placement and Cost

Many flight attendants have logistical complications to work out through treatment including, filing for leave of absence, determining the sources of funding to cover the cost of treatment (e.g., health insurance, disability programs, Medicaid, and family financial resources), and determining where to get treatment All logistical requirements advancing the flight attendant from the referral phase to actual placement at a treatment facility are primarily managed by the FADAP peer program.

A typical treatment episode includes a detox phase (as needed), psychiatric evaluation, medical evaluation, a 28–30-day residential treatment episode (which may include individual and group therapy, family treatment, substance abuse education, and trauma-specific interventions), with step-downs to a partial hospitalization program and/or intensive outpatient program, followed by an outpatient program as needed.[29] FADAP supports the use of therapeutic medications that are nonaddictive.[30] The use of medication-assisted treatment is also supported by FADAP for detoxification but not as maintenance medications. FADAP supports an abstinence model for flight attendants returning to safety-sensitive duties.

According to FADAP staff, based on a random survey they conducted among peer programs at various airlines, the ratio of residential treatment placements to nonresidential and peer support is 1:3.[31] That means, for

---

[28]FADAP's *2021 Annual Report* was provided by FADAP to the committee for review but is not available for the public.

[29]FADAP staff response to the committee-issued questionnaire, August 2022.

[30]Ibid.

[31]Ibid.

every one flight attendant placed in a FADAP-approved residential treatment program, three flight attendants received some other form of peer assistance, engaged in mutual help groups (MHGs) and/or clinical intervention initiated at any of these levels of care: partial hospital outpatient program, intensive outpatient program (IOP), or standard outpatient care.

FADAP does not pay for any treatment services. The level of care provided to a flight attendant is typically limited to what is authorized by the flight attendant's health insurance, or to the extent of what the flight attendant's personal financial resources can cover. For those without insurance, FADAP will refer the flight attendant into sliding-fee-scale programs or assist in applying for Medicaid. Two notable exceptions, however, were cited by the FADAP staff. One airline covers 100 percent of the treatment cost, including deductibles and out-of-pocket costs, for flight attendants placed in a 30-day residential treatment in a FADAP-approved treatment facility. At another airline, an automatic authorization for 28–30 residential days is provided to flight attendants placed by FADAP peers into health insurance-covered and FADAP-approved residential treatment programs.

Per FADAP staff estimates, the allowable rate per day ranges from $600 to $900 in a residential facility, $450 to $650 in a partial hospital outpatient program, and $250 to $350 in an IOP. The staff cited in their response to the committee's FADAP questionnaire that between 2019 and 2021, 445 flight attendants were placed in residential treatment programs. The length of stay in these treatment programs and/or some combination with a Physician Health Program was as follows: 230 flight attendants had an average stay of 28 to 39 days; 158 spent 40 to 60 days; 46 spent 60-plus days; and 11 were discharged before treatment completion.

Progress in the flight attendant's treatment is reported, with a release of information in place, by the treatment provider on a weekly basis to the assigned FADAP peer case manager and to the FADAP staff. The information is kept confidential from external agencies such as the FAA and from the employer (airline), unless a release of information is signed by the flight attendant.

The FADAP peer case manager performs other support activities while the flight attendant is in treatment. This includes contacting and scheduling family member participation in a family treatment program, coordinating and participating in the flight attendant's continuing care and discharge planning, and selecting mentors from a list provided by the FADAP staff to be paired with flight attendants as they transition out of primary treatment.

A mentor is a flight attendant who self-identifies as a person in recovery from a substance use disorder has at least two years of "solid recovery," as defined by local FADAP leadership, has returned to duty, and volunteers to offer support to flight attendants coming out of treatment. A mentor's primary role is to lend a listening ear and help the flight attendant successfully navigate recovery in the first year. Unlike peers, mentors are not given formal training to be a part of the recovery process. A mentor is not the same as the sponsor for a 12-step support program.

Continuing Care Services and Recovery Support

After discharge from treatment, the assigned volunteer peer case manager conducts a series of follow-up activities on a periodic basis—within 24 hours of discharge, weekly for the first 12 weeks after discharge, every two weeks for months 3 to 6, and monthly from months 6 to 12.[32] The purpose of these follow-up contacts is to ensure that the continuing care plan provided at discharge is being followed to maintain the flight attendant's wellness in the first year of recovery.

The recovery support services include, among others:

- 12-step support, such as through Wings of Sobriety;
- flight attendant family education classes and educational materials;
- resource materials on flying and medication (available on the FADAP website);
- wearing FADAP recovery pins; and
- mentorship program for flight attendant in recovery.

Employee Return-to-Duty Procedure

Determining the fitness for duty of nonmedically certified transportation safety-sensitive employees usually follows a process spelled out in collective bargaining agreements between the company and the union. Since flight attendants are not required to be medically certified, there are no FAA required tests or evaluations. A provider's release note is all that is required.

If the flight attendant was referred to FADAP due to a positive DOT test result, the DOT return-to-duty process is followed, depending on the airline regulation. The process includes a substance-use evaluation by a qualified SAP, completion of that professional's recommended education or treatment, clearance by the SAP to return to flight attendant duties, and a negative result on a return-to-duty drug/alcohol test. FADAP helps the flight attendant complete this process, regardless of whether the airline regulation allows for conditional reinstatement (vs. termination).

---

[32]Ibid.

Program Monitoring and Outcomes Measurement

The overall program performance is monitored by the FAA contractor, AFA-CWA.[33] AFA-CWA does not monitor individual cases or engage in flight attendant testing on a routine basis. The airline or union that sponsors the FADAP peer program has oversight responsibility only for the support and follow-up activities that they provide to facilitate treatment placement and recovery.

The FADAP tracking database was developed to quantify the effectiveness of the FADAP across airlines, and to identify possible risk factors, treatment failures, and areas for potential improvement. The database captures data only concerning flight attendants placed in a FADAP-approved residential treatment program. Flight attendants referred to intensive outpatient programs, individual therapy, or MHGs who may have received peer assistance are not reported in the database. The tracked data are analyzed and reported to the FADAP Advisory Board and are presented to the airlines, unions, and flight attendant leaders while maintaining the confidentiality and privacy of the FADAP participants. Access to the database for other research purposes is handled on a case-by-case basis.

In addition to the administrative and clinical data maintained in the database, a follow-up survey is conducted that includes satisfaction questions on the FADAP peer program and the treatment facility (recently added). Surveys are mailed or emailed to flight attendants one year after the initial treatment episode. In 2020, a new survey was introduced with a shorter timeframe (after three to four weeks post treatment). This new survey includes survey items to capture intermediary outcome measures.[34]

The FADAP monitors both process and outcome measures. Some examples follow:

- Process measures:
    - primary treatment diagnosis for drug, alcohol, and mental health (using DSM-5-TR);
    - level of satisfaction with FADAP peer program, using Likert scale questionnaire;
    - level of satisfaction with treatment provider, using Likert scale questionnaire;
    - treatment engagement, using Likert scale questionnaire (rated by both the treatment provider and the flight attendant); and
    - number of treatment episodes for the flight attendant.

---

[33] Ibid.

[34] "Workplace Outcomes Related to Participation" in the FADAP *2021 Annual Report*.

- Workplace outcomes:
  —work engagement;
  —presenteeism;
  —lost work time;
  —workplace behavior such as flight attendant's reported improvement in attendance, drinking past cut-off time, showing up for a flight hung-over, not showing up for a trip due to substance use, and self-perspective on overall work performance; and
  —return on investment measured by the flight attendant's reported (a) adherence to safety procedures and compliance with FAA and company policies; (b) rapport with management, coworkers, and customers; and (c) professionalism, presenteeism, and reliability.

FADAP Summary

While in-depth analysis is covered in Chapter Five, some general observations can be made about FADAP's model for treatment referral and recovery support as it offers a framework in which unpaid peers play an essential role in the flight attendant's decision to seek treatment, be engaged in treatment, and have a successful journey to recovery for a safe return to duty. However, a more proactive effort in secondary and tertiary prevention through early identification and intervention, rather than waiting until the flight attendant is "ready," may encourage more flight attendants to seek support and treatment earlier. Additionally, FADAP can improve its process by adopting a more individualized approach to treatment and recovery; level of care and length of stay should be individualized to the flight attendant's unique circumstances based on thorough assessment using the American Society of Addiction Medicine dimensions. Most importantly, consideration to address the likely program challenges discussed below may strengthen the program.

Limited Funding Sources for Treatment

Flight attendants can still incur significant costs regardless of level of care. Additionally, the decision of a flight attendant to enter treatment goes beyond the actual expenses incurred in treatment. Their absence from work while in treatment leads to loss in income for many flight attendants. Furthermore, the type and length of treatment depend heavily on what services are covered by the flight attendant's health insurance, which in turn differs from airline to airline. Expenses associated with treatment may impact a flight attendant's decision to pursue or delay treatment.

Heavy Reliance on Peer Volunteers

Heavy reliance on volunteers to support the FADAP peer model could result in a less efficient program if there is a decline in the number of volunteers, both for trained peers and mentors. This could disrupt the program's ability to maintain effective operations. It may be essential for FADAP to have a program continuity plan by incentivizing enrollment of peers and mentors rather than relying on volunteers. FADAP may also consider establishing the efficacy of its peer-support model in collaboration with ongoing support from professionals in the field and by examining the evidence base to further explore how benefits could be maximized from a peer intervention or support model.

Data Collection and Data Analysis

Using data from flight attendants' FADAP intake and follow-up forms, the FADAP central office maintains a database. This database is used to track program-level outcomes for flight attendants who engage in residential treatment. De-identified data from this database were provided to the study committee, which found numerous issues with the data. The population covered in the FADAP database is limited only to flight attendants who received treatment from FADAP-approved residential treatment programs, and there is a high degree of missingness. Therefore, the database does not capture all of FADAP peer interactions with flight attendants. Flight attendants who received services through nonresidential treatment and peer support (e.g., intensive outpatient, outpatient, individual therapy, MHGs) are currently not reported. Also, only 19 of the 24 peer programs at individual airlines report data to the FADAP database. On this basis, it is difficult to ascertain the prevalence of flight attendants engaging in substance misuse, those needing substance use treatment, and the corresponding treated population.

In addition, FADAP conducted follow-up surveys 12 months after initial treatment. This timeframe potentially presents recall bias, and it shows a high degree of loss to follow-up. Because there are few paired pre-post surveys in the dataset, arguments on program effectiveness and outcomes based on these data may be unreliable. A more meaningful data collection protocol and robust analysis of the data are needed to develop stronger arguments for program improvement and decision support.

3

Evidence-Based Practices for Identifying and Treating Substance Use Disorders

With a wealth of new research, a robust evidence base has emerged over the past few decades that can now be applied to better support people with substance use disorders. This chapter presents the state of current knowledge about the use of substances and progression to severe substance use disorders for the general population, highlighting the shift in thinking in which professionals have adopted a disease model of addiction and increasingly apply prevention frameworks to substance use disorders. The chapter also points to key elements of screening, assessment, and treatment of substance use disorders, including medication-assisted treatment (MAT) and ongoing health monitoring. Lastly, given the lack of high-quality studies of treatment outcomes specifically among professionals in safety-sensitive industries, the chapter summarizes evidence-supported practices for treatment with special attention to applying the indirect, but still valuable, research findings for professionals in safety-sensitive occupations, including pilots and flight attendants.

OVERVIEW OF SUBSTANCE USE DISORDERS

Substance use is common in the United States across all demographic groups. Most people typically first experiment with substances that have addiction potential prior to the age of 18 (Schramm-Sapyta et al., 2009). The heaviest use of these substances often occurs between adolescence and young adulthood and generally decreases following young adulthood. Most individuals who experiment with substances do not develop a substance use disorder, and the majority of those who do develop a disorder experience mild to moderate disorders. Those at highest risk of developing a substance use disorder have "earlier onset of use, history of traumatic events, family history of substance use, and/or mental health problems" (McLellan et al., 2022). Once the problem has progressed to a severe substance use disorder—the point at which substance use becomes a chronic, relapsing condition—it is often referred to as addiction.

Notably, alcohol is the most used and misused substance in the United States and across much of the world (Sudhinaraset et al., 2016; Substance Abuse Center for Behavioral Health Statistics and Quality, 2023). The data are clear that use at a younger age and a pattern of binge drinking are associated with increased risk of developing an alcohol use disorder (Hingson et al., 2006; Sudhinaraset et al., 2016; Substance Abuse Center for Behavioral Health Statistics and Quality, 2023). The National Institute on Alcohol Abuse and Alcoholism (NIAAA) has developed research-based guidelines (see Figure 3-1 and Table 3-1) to help identify high-risk drinking patterns in adults that may lead to substance-use disorders. Alcohol usage becomes high-risk when men consume more than four drinks on any day or more than 14 drinks per week, while for women the prescribed limits are no more than three drinks on any day or more than seven drinks per week (NIAAA, 2020).[1]

However, newer research completed by the World Health Organization (WHO) suggests that no safe amount of alcohol consumption exists, and that while NIAAA guidelines provide insight for those with high-risk drinking patterns that may progress to a disorder, they do not accurately reflect the health risk of even relatively low levels of alcohol consumption for the general public (Manthey & Rehm, 2022; World Health Organization, 2023).

People with substance use problems underreport their use and generally lack insight into the severity of their disease (Bone et al., 2016; Delaney-Black et al., 2010). These traits are exacerbated when a person is entering treatment in response to a problem at work, at the requirement of their employer, or at the requirement of a professional monitoring organization (Vayr et al., 2019; Wooley et al., 2013). By the time a substance use problem presents within a work setting, the disease has typically progressed to a severe level. Professional identity can be paramount for safety-sensitive professionals, and they work hard to maintain their reputation for competence and control (DeHoff & Cusick, 2018), generally while masking even acceptable forms of struggle within our culture (e.g., raising children, work stressors, divorce). Commonly, professionals in these situations engage in positive impression management, attempting to control how they are perceived, highlighting their strengths, and downplaying any problems (Brown

---

[1]After a prepublication version of the report was released, generalized key messages from a table were converted to text to mitigate any potential copyright concerns.

HOW MUCH IS TOO MUCH?

WHAT'S A "STANDARD DRINK"?

In the United States, a "standard drink" (also known as an alcoholic drink-equivalent) is defined as any beverage containing 0.6 fluid ounces or 14 grams of pure alcohol. Although the drinks pictured here are different sizes, each contains approximately the same amount of alcohol and counts as one U.S. standard drink or one alcoholic drink equivalent.

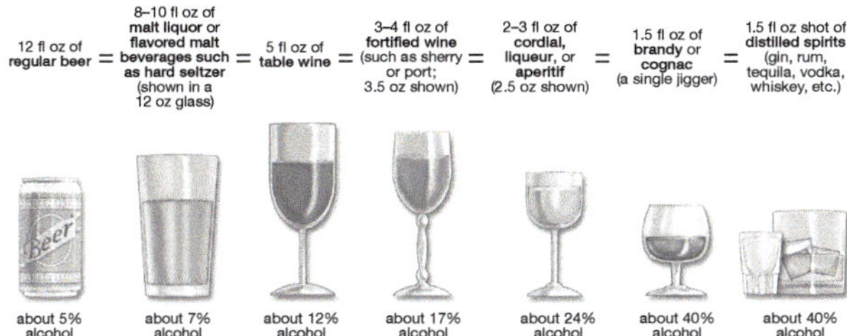

Each drink shown above represents one U.S. standard drink and has an equivalent amount (0.6 fluid ounces) of "pure" ethanol. Each beverage portrayed above represents one standard drink (or one alcoholic drink equivalent), defined in the United States as any beverage containing 0.6 fl oz or 14 grams of pure alcohol. The percentage of pure alcohol, expressed here as alcohol by volume (alc/vol), varies within and across beverage types. Although the standard drink amounts are helpful for following health guidelines, they may not reflect customary serving sizes.

HOW MANY DRINKS ARE IN COMMON CONTAINERS?

The table below shows the approximate number of standard drinks (or alcoholic drink equivalents) found in common containers.

regular beer (5% alc/vol)	malt liquor (7% alc/vol)	table wine (12% alc/vol)	80-proof distilled spirits (40% alc/vol)
12 fl oz = 1	12 fl oz = 1½	750 ml (a regular wine bottle) = 5	a shot (1.5 oz glass/50 ml bottle) = 1
16 fl oz = 1⅓	16 fl oz = 2		a mixed drink or cocktail = 1 or more
22 fl oz = 2	22 fl oz = 2½		200 ml (a "half pint") = 4½
40 fl oz = 3⅓	40 fl oz = 4½		375 ml (a "pint" or "half bottle") = 8½
			750 ml (a "fifth") = 17

FIGURE 3-1 How much is too much?
SOURCE: National Institute on Alcohol Abuse and Alcoholism, n.d.

TABLE 3-1 Heavy Alcohol Use for Men and Women[a]

	MEN	WOMEN
Drink on a single day	5 or more	4 or more
	AND	**AND**
Drinks per week	15 or more	8 or more

NOTE: [a]After a prepublication version of the report was released, this table was changed to reflect the source information more accurately.
SOURCE: Data from NIAAA (https://www.niaaa.nih.gov/alcohol-health/overview-alcohol-consumption/moderate-binge-drinking)

et al., 2015; Picard et al., 2023). Individuals with severe substance use disorders seek opportunities to use substances; professionals with substance use disorders may obtain positions or shifts that allow them to hide their disease (e.g., working overnight shifts, flying with smaller airlines with less oversight, turning down social time to hide their drinking).

As noted in Chapter 1, literature discussing substance use disorders among pilots and flight attendants suggests that they may experience rates of illness like those in the general population, though there is little validated data to directly support this. (Porges, 2013). However, of the more than 41 million adults in need of substance use disorder treatment, just under two percent received any type of treatment within the past year (SAMHSA, 2022). Most individuals (~97%) with a substance use disorder believe they *do not need* treatment, a small percentage (~2%) believe they need treatment but *did not seek* treatment in the past year, and only a fraction (~1%) *made an effort* to receive treatment (SAMHSA, 2022a).

Engaging in treatment for substance use disorders is associated with significant reductions in substance use, along with improvement in overall health and quality of life (Lail & Fairbairn, 2018; McLellan et al., 2000). However, the effectiveness of these approaches is substantially hampered by poor adherence. Though effectiveness varies significantly by treatment type, it is generally estimated that less than half of those who initiate substance use disorder treatment will still be abstinent a year later (Gaudiano et al., 2011; Milward et al., 2014; Moos et al., 1999; Sliedrecht et al., 2019). Even in physician health programs, with physicians representing a safety-sensitive group, relapse rates over five years can be 22 percent (Dupont & Merlo, 2018).

The literature has revealed several variables associated with retention in treatment and therapeutic success. These include patient characteristics such as engagement in the treatment process (e.g., compliance with medication, adherence to appointments), sociodemographic variables (e.g., age), clinical history (e.g., substance use disorder severity and concomitant psychiatric diagnosis), psychosocial characteristics (e.g., motivation), and neuropsychological variables (e.g., inhibitory control).

Following the identification of the substance use disorder and referral to treatment, people in safety-sensitive populations, which includes those working in construction, transportation, and healthcare, are removed from their positions and are unable to return to work until they complete all return-to-work requirements. These requirements often include completion of treatment, substance use abstinence, and a fitness-for-duty assessment. Rates of alcohol and other substance misuse among pilots and flight attendants have been shown to be potentially comparable to the rates among other skilled professionals and safety-sensitive populations (Atherton, 2019; Horton et al., 2011). There is also evidence that the occurrence of substance use among pilots involved in civil aviation accidents is similar to that found in the non-flying public (Botch & Johnson, 2009). Furthermore, findings from the National Transportation Safety Board (2020) suggest that misuse of licit and illicit substances among pilots is increasing.

Early detection and intervention have been shown to be important factors in the successful management of substance use disorders, reducing symptom severity and facilitating a more rapid return to full functioning. Thus, screening for substance use and mental health problems is recommended by various major health organizations (U.S. Preventive Services Task Force, 2018; White, 2012). Though data on treatment retention and success are lacking, specifically among safety-sensitive professionals, there are data to suggest that workplace-supported recovery is associated with positive outcomes regarding both drug use and employment (DeFulio et al., 2009; Frone et al., 2022). Therefore, when correctly implemented, programs such as the Human Intervention Motivational Study and Flight Attendant Drug and Alcohol Program (FADAP) have the potential to successfully manage substance use disorders and ensure a return to work among their respective safety-sensitive populations.

Diagnostic Criteria for Substance Use Disorders

Prior to the adoption of scientific, medical models of addiction, people with substance use disorders were viewed as lacking moral character, and the condition of addiction was viewed as a choice. As a result, the response to people with substance use disorders was punitive. More current models of addiction view it as a brain disease. Health care professionals determine whether someone meets criteria for a substance use disorder using the *Diagnostic and Statistical Manual of Mental Disorders* (DSM), the authoritative guide for diagnosing mental disorders (see Box 3-1 for the more recently adopted disease model of addiction).

The current version of the diagnostic manual, the DSM-5,[2] revised the DSM-IV by eliminating the diagnostic categories of "substance abuse" and "substance dependence." Not only is the term "substance abuse" stigmatizing, but the DSM-IV abuse criteria lacked reliability and validity (Hasin et al., 2013). The DSM-IV term "substance dependence" created confusion with certain prescribed medications that were beneficial but were nonetheless associated with physiological dependence symptoms, such as withdrawal symptoms upon abrupt discontinuation.

---

[2]For report consistency and readability, the committee is using "DSM-5" instead of "DSM-5 (text revision)," but readers should update their best practices as new additions of DSM are released.

BOX 3-1
Disease Model of Addiction

The view of addiction as a moral failing historically discouraged people from focusing on prevention and treatment, while it exacerbated stigma. The American Medical Association classified *alcoholism* as a disease in 1956 and included *drug addiction* as a disease in 1987. This classification of addiction as a medical illness was reinforced by an influential analysis that compared addiction with other chronic medical conditions including diabetes, hypertension, and asthma (McLellan et al., 2000). That analysis found similar impacts of hereditary and environmental factors in both addiction and these other chronic medical conditions. Furthermore, it found similar treatment response rates and relapse rates in all these illnesses, all of which required behavioral change as a part of treatment adherence. In brief, this newer brain disease model recognizes that changes in the brain not only occur in response to acute exposure to alcohol and drugs but can also persist long after an individual stops regular use (Leshner, 1997). This shift in perspective has led to treatment and policy advances while also beginning to destigmatize the illness and considering psychosocial factors that play a role in the progression to more severe disease (Heilig et al., 2021; Volkow & Koob, 2015; Volkow et al., 2016).

While the consequences of addiction often put others' lives in danger in ways that diabetes, asthma, and hypertension do not (e.g., driving under the influence, stealing to obtain money to buy substance), treatment is as effective for substance use disorders as it is for these other chronic conditions. When treatment is provided to people with substance use disorders, a significant decline in criminal behavior and in financial cost to society is observed.

SOURCE: Data from Hellig et al., 2021; Volkow & Koob, 2015; Volkow et al., 2016).

The criteria for substance use disorder cited in the DSM-5 (American Psychiatric Association, 2022) include 11 symptoms that broadly describe four pathological patterns of substance use (rephrased below):

1. Impaired control over substance use, including:[3]
   a. Using the substance more, or longer, than intended

---

[3]After a prepublication version of the report was released, information from a figure was integrated into the following text due to copyright considerations.

    b.   More than a single instance of unsuccessfully attempting to reduce or stop using the substance

    c.   Experiencing strong cravings to use a substance that disrupt the ability to think about other things

2. Impairment in social functioning, including:
    a.   Excessive time using or being sick from the substance or its after effects
    b.   Interference in executing home, family, school, or professional responsibilities due to substance use
    c.   Continued substance use despite negative impacts to personal relationships
    d.   Reducing or withdrawing from activities of interest due to substance use

3. Recurrent substance use which puts the person using the substance at risk for physical and psychological harm, including:
    a.   Getting into dangerous situations due to substance use
    b.   Continued substance use despite deleterious mental health outcomes

4. Pharmacological criteria of tolerance and withdrawal, including:
    a.   Having to use more of the substance to achieve desired effects
    b.   Feeling negative physical and mental symptoms related to withdrawal

In formalizing a diagnosis, the number of symptoms determines the severity of the disease (e.g., 2 or 3 symptoms = mild; 4 or 5 symptoms = moderate; 6+ symptoms = severe). Notably, neither the quantity of substance used nor blood alcohol levels are features of the diagnostic criteria. For example, the amount of alcohol consumed on an average day or the blood alcohol content (BAC) at a given time (e.g., DUI) are not factors in determining whether a person has a substance use disorder.

The diagnostic criteria for substance use disorders apply to all substances with addictive potential. However, the diagnoses are differentiated by substance in regard to symptoms of intoxication and withdrawal. For example, withdrawal from alcohol and stimulants, such as cocaine, may result in sleep difficulties and agitation; however, withdrawal from alcohol can also result in vomiting, hallucinations, and seizures, whereas withdrawal from stimulants can result in a dysphoric mood, fatigue, and increased appetite. The terms "addiction" and "alcoholism" are regularly used by people with substance use disorders; however, DSM-5 does not use these terms because of their "uncertain definition and potentially negative connotation" (APA, 2022) The DSM-5 does recognize that some clinicians will use the term "addiction" to refer to severe substance use disorders.

While diagnostic criteria for substance use disorders as defined by the DSM-5 apply to all people, the Federal Aviation Administration (FAA) uses different definitions to determine when a pilot has a problem. For example, as reviewed in Chapter 2 of this report, the blood alcohol concentration limit for pilots *reporting to duty* is 0.04. This lower threshold than the 0.08 for the average American car driver is to protect the public from harm as research has shown impairment occurring at even lower levels of blood alcohol concentration (Mumenthaler et al., 2003; NHTSA, 2000). Further, while this is not written into policy, it is widely accepted by aviation medical examiners (AMEs) and encouraged at the Human Intervention Motivational Study (HIMS) conference to consider a blood alcohol content at time of DUI or reporting to duty of 0.15–0.199 as an indication of reaching the FAA definition of abuse and a blood alcohol content of 0.2 or higher as the FAA definition of dependence. This stricter threshold is to protect the public and impairment has been demonstrated to affect drivers having lower levels of blood alcohol concentration (NHTSA, 2000). Pilots and flight attendants employed by larger airlines are more likely to have treatment costs covered regardless of received diagnoses. However, pilots at smaller and mid-sized airlines could meet the FAA definition of substance abuse or dependence but not qualify for insurance coverage, as they would not have a diagnosis based on the clinical DSM-5 criteria for a substance use disorder.

Benefits of Prevention and Early Intervention

The costs of not addressing substance misuse and substance use disorders can go beyond the individual consequences, with substance misuse across this continuum resulting in costs to society at large of more than $400 billion annually (Murthy, 2017). Substance misuse increases company healthcare costs, missed work days, injuries on the job, and rates of employee turnover, while it decreases productivity. Too commonly, intervention efforts in the workplace focus on the most severe cases of substance use disorders, but the consequences of mild to moderate substance use disorders (i.e., two to five DSM-5 symptoms) account for more societal substance-related harms than severe substance use disorders (i.e., six or more DSM-5 symptoms; McClellan et al., 2022). Unfortunately, substance use and work are intimately intertwined, regardless of whether use occurs at work. The concept of *pre-addiction*, defined as mild to moderate substance use disorders, has been proposed as a crucial point for intervention that is analogous to the care model of diabetes in which prediabetes is a crucial point for intervention (McClellan et al., 2022). Investment in identifying at-risk employees and treatment could result in savings for both the company and society in general by stopping the progression of the disorder. In fact, it is estimated that every dollar spent on substance use disorder treatment saves four dollars in healthcare costs (Murthy, 2016). Professionals with substance use disorders in safety-sensitive occupations pose a greater risk to others and cost to society because of the nature of their work; as a result, the workplace can be an ideal point for intervention.

DISEASE PREVENTION

Recognizing that addiction is a disease and not a moral failing, focus and investment can be made to strategically optimize outcomes and have the most impact. A disease prevention model highlights the different components to address the disease, including health promotion, prevention, treatment, and recovery (see Figure 3-2). The Substance Abuse and Mental Health Services Administration (SAMHSA) defines prevention as being "delivered prior to the onset of a disorder. These interventions are intended to prevent or reduce the risk of developing a behavioral health problem."

Integrating Approaches to Improve Care

Traditionally, services for preventing and treating substance use disorders have been delivered separately from other mental health and general healthcare services. However, it is increasingly recommended that assessment and treatment for substance misuse be integrated with other health care delivery (Murthy, 2016). This approach is a model of integrated behavioral healthcare that brings together primary care and behavioral health clinicians, such as clinical psychologists and clinical social workers,

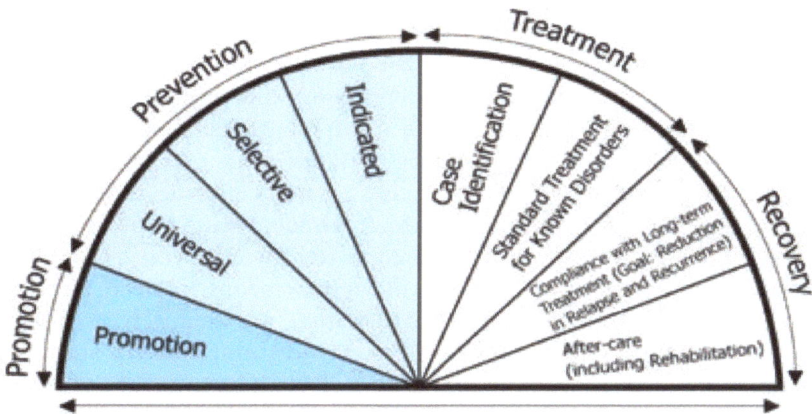

FIGURE 3-2 Disease prevention model.
SOURCE: Adapted from Haggerty & Mrazek, 1994.

to provide a team based, evidence-based approach to patient-centered care. One more integrated approach to addressing substance use is called, Screening, Brief Intervention, and Referral to Treatment (SBIRT). SBIRT is an evidence-based practice to identify, reduce, and prevent misuse of alcohol and tobacco in primary care settings; however, its strongest evidence is within the context of alcohol use (Barata et al., 2017; Mello et al., 2018). The approach is also gaining traction in the workplace, with EAPs offering a set number of free therapy sessions and wellness initiatives (McPherson et al., 2010; Taranowski & Mahieu, 2013).

The SBIRT model adapted to the workplace consists of three primary components: (1) screening employees for risky substance use behaviors using standardized screening tools; (2) a brief intervention by motivating employees to make a specific change; and (3) referral to treatment to brief therapy or additional treatment services.[4]

BEST PRACTICES IN SCREENING, ASSESSING, AND TREATING SUBSTANCE USE DISORDERS

While SBIRT is often used in primary care and emergency medicine settings, the spectrum of screening, assessment, treatment, and ongoing monitoring for substance use disorders can cross multiple environments (SAMHSA, 2022b). Evidence examining the use of SBIRT in the occupational setting is not strong, but it has still proven to be a valuable tool in general. This section highlights evidence-supported practices across that continuum, with special considerations that could be applied for safety-sensitive professionals where appropriate.

Screening

The U.S. Preventive Services Task Force recommends that primary care providers screen for anxiety, depression, alcohol use, and tobacco use in adults and offer brief behavioral interventions as indicated. Many people with substance use disorders do not seek treatment on their own due to a variety of reasons, including not believing that they need treatment, not being ready to engage in treatment, being unaware of treatment options, not knowing how to access treatment that is available, the political climate, perceived stigma of what it means to need treatment, and other social and structural barriers that are themselves linked to risks for substance use, like the cost of care, low employment status, low household income, and inadequate (or lack of housing; U.S. Preventive Services Task Force, 2018).

---

[4]For a practical example, see https://vitalalabama.com/professional-resources/sbirt-tool-kit/

People often access the healthcare system for other reasons, however, including annual physicals or other preventative care appointments, acute health problems like illness, injury, or overdose, as well as chronic health conditions such as HIV/AIDS, heart disease, diabetes, anxiety, or depression. If people access care of any kind, they most commonly reach out to a primary care provider, so screening related to substance use as part of these more general health assessments is a crucial point of prevention and intervention. If a person screens positive on measures delivered as part of these visits, follow-up assessment is indicated. The U.S. Preventive Services Task Force recommends that individuals with problematic levels of alcohol use be offered patient-centered advice about recommended limits and information on how alcohol use relates to other health conditions.

Disorders characterized by symptoms of anxiety and depression and in response to trauma often lead people to use substances to obtain some relief. Thus, screening for mental health conditions that often co-occur with substance use disorders is also particularly important. Addressing these concerns can be preventative of problematic substance use and progression from use to a severe substance use disorder. The National Institute on Drug Abuse offers several evidence-based screening and assessment tools for varying types of substance use (National Institute on Drug Abuse [NIDA], n.d.).

For pilots, the FAA requires a medical examination with a specialized AME every six months to five years, depending on their age and the type of flying they do. Part of this evaluation includes a review of diagnoses related to psychosis, bipolar disorder, severe personality disorders, and substance misuse and dependence; however, the review process varies by AME. While most public and private health programs require providers to screen for alcohol and depression, HIMS's reported 0.5 percent positive screening referral rate suggests possible inadequate attention to such screening (Snyder, 2021). Incorporation of substance use, mental health, and stress screeners could be integrated during these assessments to standardize the evaluation process and integrate a prevention strategy.

Safety-sensitive professionals are acutely aware of the consequences that a mental health or substance-related concern can have on their career. As a result, they may minimize these issues and often do not establish care with a primary care provider, avoiding regular screenings (DeHoff & Cusick, 2018). The lack of discussion around substance use can encourage silence and facilitate shame, stigma, and suffering in isolation. Screening specific to assessing when substance use started, whether the professional has a history of traumatic events or a family history of substance misuse, and any mental health problems can help identify safety-sensitive professionals at high risk of developing a substance use disorder. If employee screening does not adequately identify safety-sensitive professionals at risk of developing a substance use disorder, the benefit of professional substance use programs is fundamentally weak.

Based on that screening, which includes assessment for co-occurring substance use and mental health disorders, a determination is made about what support the client may need. Brief intervention includes five steps: (1) asking permission to discuss the screening results; (2) reviewing the screening results or substance use patterns and providing feedback; (3) exploring how the presenting problem may be related to substance use and how the employee views the identified problem; (4) assessing and negotiating readiness to change and developing a plan with the employee to achieve goals; and (5) discussing next steps, which could include brief treatment. Finally, clients who require treatment beyond the brief intervention could then be referred to options within the structure of their respective program.[5]

Evidence examining the use of SBIRT in the occupational setting is not strong, but it has still proven to be a valuable tool in general.

Assessment of Substance Use Disorders

Assessment is a crucial step for determining the severity of a person's substance misuse problem, identifying whether they have a substance use disorder and any co-occurring conditions, and making recommendations to address their unique needs for healing. This process allows all constituents to gain an understanding of the current situation and the most appropriate course of action. With proper releases of information (ROIs), the individual being assessed, their identified family, their employer and/or professional support program, and treatment providers can be included in this process, both for obtaining collateral information and for executing the recommendations.

It is best practice for treatment providers, whether at formal treatment centers or an individual provider, to do a thorough assessment of an individual seeking care. This process can vary significantly depending on the point of entry to care, whether from a provider in private practice, in a formal treatment facility intake, or in a more multidisciplinary assessment during residential treatment. The best assessments include collateral information (APA, 2020) to gather data beyond what is provided by the person seeking care and screen for common co-occurring disorders and factors that put someone at higher risk for developing a substance use disorder (e.g., onset of use, family history of substance use, trauma history, anxiety, depression, process addictions, physical complaints [APA, 2020]. People with substance use problems tend to underreport their use and generally can lack insight into the severity of their own disease (Halpern et al., 2019; Steinhoff et al., 2023). These issues can be amplified when entering

---

[5]Ibid.

treatment at the requirement of an employer or a professional monitoring organization due to attempts at positive impression management (Brown et al., 2015; Picard et al., 2023).

Available Models for Assessment

Two theoretical frames guide the best substance use disorder assessments: The Biopsychosocial-Spiritual Approach and the American Society of Addiction Medicine (ASAM) Criteria; both of which focus on a multidimensional approach and encourage clinically driven treatment and recommendations. The biopsychosocial model, first introduced by Engel (1977) and later expanded to include spirituality (McKee & Chappel, 1992), challenged the traditional biomedical approach to treating disease to include a more holistic approach. This model recognizes that "the biological, psychological, social, and spiritual are distinct dimensions of the person, and no one aspect can be disaggregated from the whole" (Sulmasy, 2002). Spirituality, as defined by Puchalski et al. (2009), "is the aspect of humanity that refers to the way individuals seek and express meaning and purpose, and the way they experience their connectedness to the moment, to self, to others, to nature, and to the significant or sacred." The *Alcoholics Anonymous Big Book* further supports this dimension; it describes alcohol use disorders and resentments that often accompany them as being a spiritual disease, "for we have been not only mentally and physically ill, we have been spiritually sick" (Alcoholics Anonymous, 2002) Thus, for a person to transition into a life of sustained recovery, it is important to assess each domain of the human experience to determine the unique interactions for the individual, to understand their presenting concerns and needs.

The ASAM model integrates the biopsychosocial-spiritual approach into six dimensions indicated for assessing the needs of people with substance use disorders (see Figure 3-3). Through an ASAM assessment, providers gather data about each of the six dimensions with the goal of determining the necessary level of care for each dimension, looking at both areas of strength and areas of concern. Providers with expertise in substance use disorders have specialized training, credentials, and insight into the presentation of these conditions and the needs of an individual for obtaining and sustaining recovery. Ultimately, a recommendation for level of care is made based on the data within each dimension and by considering the interaction across dimensions, along a continuum of care (see Figures 3-3 and 3-4).

Some assessments may be done before an individual seeks treatment. For example, when safety-sensitive transportation professionals violate a U.S. Department of Transportation (DOT) drug and alcohol program regulation, they are required to be evaluated by a Substance Abuse Professional (SAP). SAP credentials were developed by the DOT to assist the agency in

AT A GLANCE: THE SIX DIMENSIONS OF MULTIDIMENSIONAL ASSESSMENT

ASAM's Criteria uses six dimensions to create a holistic, biopsychosocial assessment of an individual to be used for service planning and treatment across all services and levels of care. The six dimensions are:

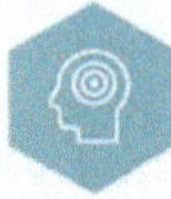

DIMENSION 1

Acute Intoxication and/or Withdrawal Potential
Exploring an individual's past and current experiences of substance use and withdrawal

DIMENSION 2

Biomedical Conditions and Complications
Exploring an individual's health history and current physical health needs

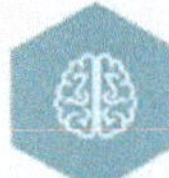

DIMENSION 3

Emotional, Behavioral, or Cognitive Conditions and Complications
Exploring an individual's mental health history and current cognitive and mental health needs

DIMENSION 4

Readiness to Change
Exploring an individual's readiness for and interest in changing

DIMENSION 5

Relapse, Continued Use or Continued Problem Potential
Exploring an individual's unique needs that influence their risk for relapse or continued use

DIMENSION 6

Recovering/Living Environment
Exploring an individual's recovery or living situation, and the people and places that can support or hinder their recovery

FIGURE 3-3 Six dimensions of multidimensional assessment.
SOURCE: Guyer et al., 2021.

FIGURE 3-4 ASAM continuum of care.
SOURCE: Guyer et al., 2021.

supporting those of its employees who were identified as having a problem with drugs or alcohol (DOT, n.d.). This credential is distinct from those mentioned above. Pilots are required to have a medical clearance to perform their job. When pilots are diagnosed with substance abuse or dependence per the FAA definitions, they lose their medical certificate to fly. To return to the cockpit, they must undergo a fitness-for-duty assessment, described below. ASAM proposes that professionals in safety-sensitive professions have four unique qualities that lead to "important and distinct" needs for assessment and treatment (see Box 3-2).

BOX 3-2
Qualities of Safety-Sensitive Professionals Leading to Important and Distinct Needs for Assessment and Treatment

People in safety-sensitive professions have a responsibility to the public. This responsibility is present both in the number of people safety-sensitive professionals interact with and the depth of impact their impairment can cause. Public trust is high for professionals in safety-sensitive occupations (e.g., law enforcement, healthcare providers, pilots, flight attendants, and other transportation roles, attorneys) and challenges that disrupt this trust can significantly impact the perception of an entire profession.

People in safety-sensitive professions benefit most from cohort-specific treatment. This therapeutic environment helps facilitate self-disclosure while decreasing shame, guilt, and stigma. Peers in similar professions can normalize the impact substance misuse and addiction have on one professionally and how it puts others at risk, while maintaining public trust in the profession.

Many professionals in safety-sensitive occupations have direct access to substances that are addictive. This includes pilots and flight attendants who have access to alcohol served on the plane.

To heal from substance use disorders, people need to assume the role of patient. Professionals in safety-sensitive occupations, particularly those in positions of significant power like pilots and customer service like flight attendants, struggle to assume the patient role. They struggle to let go of their innate caretaking, their desire to be perceived as competent, and experience difficulty in relinquishing control. Accepting help and healing requires showing up authentically and vulnerably, letting others see their suffering and accepting that they need help.

SOURCE: Data from American Society of Addiction Medicine, 2013, pp. 340–349.

In light of these unique qualities, ASAM recommends that professionals in safety-sensitive occupations discontinue work throughout the assessment period. The association further recommends that these professionals cease practice until risks to the public have been managed, all work regulations, licensure, and legal issues have been addressed, cues and triggers specific to the work environment have been identified, and a plan is in place to manage them. Further, ASAM recommends that the work environment and supervisory personnel be considerate of what it takes to sustain recovery. To be appropriate for a return to work, abstinence needs to be attained and a strong foundation of recovery established. These unique considerations add context to the assessment of these professionals. Moreover, employer policies may result in their not having income or insurance throughout this process; this added stressor often complicates the assessment.

Fitness for Duty Assessment

Most people with substance use disorders continue to work, and data suggest that work may have therapeutic effects on recovery outcomes (Frone et al., 2022; SAMHSA, 2019b; Walton & Hall, 2016). People in some safety-sensitive occupations, including pilots, will be relieved from their professional responsibilities until they complete an assessment and initial treatment and until risks to the public have been managed. As such, another unique consideration of assessing safety-sensitive professionals is the determination of fitness for duty, that is, whether and when a professional should be considered safe to return to their safety-sensitive responsibilities. While it has not been clearly defined when it is best to perform a fitness-for-duty evaluation, these evaluations would be most useful after three months of confirmed abstinence (NIDA, 2014).

In the transportation industry, many employees in safety-sensitive positions undergo fitness-for-duty assessments; pilots have more rigorous standards than most as this is required to obtain their special issuance medical certificate. The FAA defines pilot fitness for duty as "being physiologically and mentally prepared and capable of performing assigned duties at the highest degree of safety" (FAA, 2012). These assessments include psychological testing completed by a board-certified neuropsychologist and are conducted by an AME. The incorporation of psychological testing, particularly cognitive testing, provides an objective measure of functioning and impairment. If cognitive abilities have not been significantly impacted by a pilot's substance use, the pilot can be cleared to return to work after having attained sobriety, having addressed any co-occurring mental health concerns, and having demonstrated a program of recovery from illness. If cognitive impairment is present, the process for returning to work is more complicated. It may be determined that some pilots will never regain cognitive capacities to return to the cockpit; however, for others, a longer period of sustained recovery and repeat cognitive testing will be necessary to make a determination.

Treatment of Substance Use Disorders Across a Continuum of Care

The appropriate level of care for treatment and length of stay for someone with a substance use disorder is based on that individual's present clinical presentation, as understood through the biopsychosocial-spiritual model and ASAM dimensions described previously. The landscape of addiction treatment is a continuum of care ranging from Early Intervention Services (Level 0.5) to Medically Managed Intensive Inpatient Services (Level 5; see Table 3-2 below from ASAM). A person with a substance use disorder can transition between levels of care within this continuum as needed, based on the progression of their disease. Any level of care on this continuum can serve as an individual's entry point into addiction treatment, and what levels of care are available will be determined by where the person lives and their insurance plan and financial resources.

As improvement in the disease continues, the individual ideally steps down through the various levels of care; if an individual relapses or needs more support to avoid a relapse, they can step up in levels of care. Obtaining sobriety is the first step in healing. It is possible to change default neural networks, but this takes sober time, repetition, and accountability. Engaging in long-term treatment that adapts to the individual needs of each patient facilitates this healing process.

Understanding Entry into Treatment

People who need treatment for substance use disorders rarely enter treatment on their own (NIDA, 2007); but fortunately, how an individual enters treatment (e.g., voluntarily versus being mandated) does not predict whether the treatment will be beneficial (Coviello et al., 2013). People may seek treatment due to physical health problems, legal involvement, or a requirement placed on them by work or family. Members of more marginalized communities, such as African American and Latino people (Pinedo, 2019), have been found to be less likely to seek and use treatment for substance use disorders (Acevedo et al., 2018). These race-related barriers are likely due to a variety of reasons, including lack of timely access to services (Acevedo et al., 2018). For the general population, care should occur within the least restrictive environment that can appropriately address the individual's treatment needs while keeping them safe. The duration of treatment, or length of stay, should be determined by a person's progress toward their clinical treatment goals, including whether they desire

TABLE 3-2 Levels of Addiction Treatment

Level of Care	Title	Description
0.5	Early Intervention	Assessment and education for at-risk individuals who do not meet diagnostic criteria for substance use disorder
1	Outpatient Services	Less than 9 hours of service/week for recovery or motivational enhancement therapies/strategies
2.1	Intensive Outpatient Services	9 or more hours of service/week to treat multidimensional instability
2.5	Partial Hospitalization Services	20 or more hours of service/week for multidimensional instability not requiring 24-hour care
3.1	Clinically Managed Low-Intensity Residential Services	24-hour structure with available trained personnel; at least 5 hours of clinical service/week
3.3	Clinically Managed Population-Specific High-Intensity Residential Services	24-hour care with trained counselors to stabilize multidimensional imminent danger. Less intensive milieu and group treatment for those with cognitive or other impairments unable to use full active milieu or therapeutic community
3.5	Clinically Managed High-Intensity Residential Services	24-hour care with trained counselors to stabilize multidimensional imminent danger and prepare for outpatient treatment. Able to tolerate and use full active milieu or therapeutic community
3.7	Medically Monitored Intensive Inpatient Services	24-hour nursing care with physician availability for significant problems in Dimensions 1, 2, or 3; 16 hours/day of counselor availability
4	Medically Managed Intensive Inpatient Services	24-hour nursing care and daily physician care for severely unstable patients

SOURCE: Data from https://www.asam.org/asam-criteria/about-the-asam-criteria

complete abstinence or a reduction in use, not by a pre-prescribed length of a treatment program (e.g., 28- or 30-day residential program; Mee-Lee et al., 2013).

Regardless of the entry point for substance use disorder treatment, people must first be physically stabilized. Decreased use, particularly of alcohol, benzodiazepines, and opiates, can lead to significant physical symptoms. In the case of alcohol and benzodiazepines, the process of withdrawal can be life-threatening and often requires the oversight of medical providers and incorporation of MAT when people have been using long-term and/or have been using large amounts. The assessment, as described above, is important for determining what level of care is needed to safely and humanely facilitate withdrawal or plan for decreased use without exacerbating symptoms.

Importantly, withdrawal management is not sufficient treatment for substance use disorders; removing the substances from the body is often a necessary first step, yet it is not sufficient for obtaining and sustaining sobriety. Repeated withdrawal episodes can exacerbate the severity of withdrawal for people with alcohol use disorders; this is known as *kindling* (Becker, 1998). People who experience seizures as part of the detoxification process are more likely to have had repeated episodes of detox and have poorer prognosis and higher mortality rates (Becker, 1998).

Given that addiction is frequently persistent, research supports long durations of care consistent with other chronic health conditions (McClellan et al., 2000; NIDA, 2007) for best outcomes. Regardless of entry point on the continuum of care, the early phases need to provide psychoeducation and encouragement for treatment engagement. It is during these earliest days of sobriety that symptoms of co-occurring disorders may resurface with greater severity and emotions may become more intensely experienced; it may be the first time in years a person has fully experienced their guilt and shame, symptoms of anxiety, depression, and trauma without the escape of a substance. Some will experience symptoms of acute withdrawal, but for some these symptoms can persist for months as post-acute withdrawal syndrome (Bahji, 2022). These early days of treatment are particularly challenging as people often lack healthy means of coping.

Early Recovery and Maintenance Phases

Early recovery, approximately the first six weeks to three months of any level of care, should be highly structured (SAMHSA & the Office of the Surgeon General, 2006). This is necessary to shift behavioral default networks, that is, to shift from using substances to cope to using new, healthier, substance-free behaviors for recovery. Patients are supported in identifying their own triggers to use and implementing coping strategies to sustain abstinence. They are encouraged to connect with sober mutual-support communities, and also may benefit from external accountability, such as random drug and alcohol testing. Few studies have examined whether drug testing improves treatment outcomes, but some evidence suggests workplace drug testing is associated with reductions in substance use and reductions in occupational injuries (Sheridan & Winkler, 1989). Further, ASAM expert consensus is that drug testing can be useful during and after treatment to improve treatment outcomes (Jarvis et al., 2017).

The maintenance phase of treatment continues to build on early recovery. The goal of abstinence remains the same, and implementation of relapse-prevention skills and ongoing care for co-occurring conditions (i.e., in the physical, emotional, behavioral, cognitive, social, and spiritual domains) continues. People with substance use disorders and a goal of complete abstinence broaden their social support networks, build a "life worth living," and continue to address co-occurring conditions. Their bodies continue to recalibrate to a life without substances and they become more easily able to implement healthy coping skills and grow better at recognizing and tolerating the experience of urges and cravings without relapse. If a relapse occurs, it provides insight into areas the individual has not yet adequately addressed for sustaining long-term recovery and might indicate the need for a higher level of treatment.

The final stage of treatment as outlined by SAMHSA is the stage of community support (SAMHSA, 2006). While the goal of abstinence remains, the individual leans more on their community of support and distances themselves from formal treatment settings. A relapse may indicate the need to return to a more formalized level of clinical support within the continuum of care.

Transitions to a lower level of care create important opportunities for communication and collaboration between treatment providers, the patient, and their support network. While transitions may be times to celebrate the progress made, they can also be times when the risk of relapse is high if the level of support shifts too quickly. A detailed discharge plan that addresses each domain of the ASAM criteria can help facilitate a smooth transition between levels of care. It is also important to be mindful that too many aspects of a person's life are not shifting at the same time. For example, patients who transition to a lower level of care at the same time that medication changes are happening or who are leaving a sober living environment often struggle to maintain sobriety. At all levels of care, the treatment, discharge planning, therapy goals, and safety planning must be individualized to the patient and their unique needs based on multidimensional assessments. Incorporation of identified family and comprehensive discharge planning further improves outcomes.

It is difficult to make generalizations about the effectiveness of addiction treatment based on the literature, due to many challenges and variables: unique populations studied (e.g., people with alcohol use disorders vs. people with opioid use disorders); unique treatment conditions (e.g., high fidelity to treatment interventions by study clinicians vs. treatment as usual in nonresearch populations); different treatment outcomes (e.g., reduction in use vs. abstinence from use, self-report vs. objective measures); and different follow-up periods (e.g., months into treatment vs. months or years after treatment; Fleury et al., 2016). One estimate is that 40 to 60 percent of patients treated for substance use disorders are abstinent at one year after treatment (McLellan et al., 2000). However, there is considerable variability in estimates. Research has shown that both person factors and treatment factors affect treatment outcomes. For example, people with less severe substance use disorder, less psychiatric comorbidity, higher readiness to change, more social support, positive social context (employment, higher socioeconomic status, greater education), and more purpose in life tend to show better treatment outcomes (Sliedrecht et al., 2019).

There are few high-quality studies of treatment outcomes among professionals in safety-sensitive industries. A number of peer-reviewed articles have been published on chart reviews of physicians receiving substance use treatment through Physician Health Programs (PHPs). These articles document that approximately 80 percent of the physicians followed over five years of intensive monitoring showed no positive alcohol or drug test results (Dupont et al., 2009; McLellan et al., 2008). One claim is that these high success rates are attributable to the PHP care management model, as opposed to "person" factors such as physicians' high intelligence and financial resources (Dupont & Merlo, 2018). However, little is known about the specific reasons underlying the reported high success rates of this model (Merlo et al., 2022). Importantly, all PHPs may not be equal. Claims have been made about the questionable quality of some PHPs which vary across states (Lenzer, 2016). Some of the concerns include lack of documented criteria for selecting treatment centers and lack of objectivity in evaluation of physicians' need for substance use treatment, culminating in calls for regular audits (Lenzer, 2016).

MAT

MAT has been demonstrated to improve the outcome of treatment and, in the case of opioid use disorder, it is considered essential and lifesaving (Wakeman, 2017).

At all levels of care, the consensus position of substance use treatment professionals is that treatment plans should include the option for MAT for people seeking abstinence from alcohol, opioids, or tobacco.[6] Treatment providers and centers not offering this form of support are restricting

---

[6]Although there is substantial evidence for medications to treat co-occurring psychiatric illness in people with substance use disorders and evidence that the treatment of co-occurring disorders improves addiction treatment outcomes, this report will not examine this important aspect of medication as the FAA has a separate program for mental illness-related medication (for more information, see https://www.faa.gov/ame_guide/app_process/exam_tech/item47/amd/antidepressants). The main focus in this section will be on MAT for alcohol use disorders and for opioid use disorders. A detailed overview of available medications for tobacco cessation is available at: https://www.hhs.gov/sites/default/files/2020-cessation-sgr-full-report.pdf

life-saving care and denying FDA-approved medication. Rates of relapse and overdose are significantly decreased by the integration of these medications in conjunction with the continuum of therapeutic addiction care. MAT improves long-term recovery outcomes and can prevent overdose. However, as discussed in later sections, there are special considerations for the use of some of these medications by safety-sensitive professionals.

Medications for the Treatment of Alcohol Use Disorders

Three FDA-approved medications for the treatment of alcohol use disorders are currently available: disulfiram, naltrexone, and acamprosate. Disulfiram, which results in toxicity if alcohol is consumed, should only be prescribed for patients who wish to achieve complete abstinence and understand the risk of using alcohol while taking disulfiram. There is evidence from multiple studies that it works best when its administration can be monitored (Skinner et al., 2014).

Naltrexone is an opioid receptor antagonist that has been shown to be effective in the treatment of both opioid and alcohol use disorders. Naltrexone administration has been associated with greater likelihood of alcohol abstinence, fewer drinking days in those who are not abstinent, and a reduction in alcohol craving (O'Malley, 1996). Naltrexone is available as an oral medication, which may be taken daily and as a depot injection administered monthly.

Acamprosate's effectiveness was established in Europe, where it was typically prescribed after a period of alcohol abstinence. Although it is generally well tolerated, it requires oral administration every eight hours, making treatment adherence more difficult. In a meta-analysis comparing trials of acamprosate with trials of naltrexone, acamprosate was found to be slightly more efficacious in promoting abstinence and naltrexone slightly more efficacious in reducing heavy drinking and craving (Bouza et al., 2004).

Medications for the Treatment of Opioid Use Disorders

Three FDA-approved medications for the treatment of opioid use disorders are currently available: methadone, buprenorphine, and naltrexone. Methadone is an opioid receptor agonist medication and is a Schedule II drug under the Controlled Substances Act. Although methadone is often described as "controversial" and has been criticized and stigmatized as a treatment that "trades one addiction for another," there is good evidence that methadone improves a wide variety of outcomes related to opioid use disorder and that continued improvements are seen as duration of treatment with methadone lengthens (Castells et al., 2009; Connock et al.,

2007; Lim et al., 2023). Methadone is considered an "essential" medication by the WHO, and its use within the United States has occurred almost exclusively in a system of federal and state licensed and regulated Opioid Treatment Programs (OTPs). These regulations prescribe many aspects of treatment such as the need for daily attendance by patients and medication doses allowed in treatment. It is illegal for methadone to be prescribed for the treatment of an opioid use disorder outside of an OTP. It is legal for methadone to be prescribed without such oversight for pain relief, although deaths due to methadone overdose have been more frequent in people receiving methadone for pain than in those who receive it for opioid use disorder (Jones et al., 2016). Professional medical organizations have advocated for greater flexibility in the regulation of methadone treatment for opioid use disorder, because it is safe and effective when prescribed by knowledgeable professionals and because the current treatment system is difficult for patients to access and navigate.

Buprenorphine is a partial agonist at the mu opioid receptor. As with methadone, it is considered an essential medication by the WHO. Whereas methadone is a Schedule II drug under the Controlled Substances Act, buprenorphine is a Schedule III drug, which means it is seen as a drug with less misuse potential. This Schedule III status was important in permitting its prescription in individual office-based practices rather than OTPs, although OTPs are permitted to dispense buprenorphine. The 2000 Drug Addiction Treatment Act allowed physicians to use buprenorphine to treat patients at their office rather than only in an OTP. A mandatory educational requirement, "the X-waiver" was established as part of the act. However, due to the safety and effectiveness of buprenorphine and the need for more available buprenorphine in attempts to reduce deaths from opioid overdose, the need for this waiver was eliminated in 2023. Buprenorphine and methadone seem to have equivalent efficacy in the treatment of opioid use disorder (Lim et al., 2022; Mattick et al., 2014; West et al., 2000), though methadone is associated with better treatment retention.[7] Buprenorphine is now available as an extended-release, monthly subcutaneous injection that can enhance treatment adherence.

Naltrexone is a mu opioid receptor antagonist. Initial trials of oral naltrexone for the treatment of opioid use disorder were disappointing because of poor treatment adherence in treated populations (Minozzi et al., 2011). The availability of a depot form of naltrexone that can be given as a monthly injection, although originally developed for the treatment of alcohol use disorder, was recognized as an important potential treatment

---

[7]The citations are consistent with prior data, but there is a growing clinical sense that individuals using fentanyl are treated more effectively with methadone than buprenorphine, in the professional experience of some committee members.

modality for opioid use disorder. The efficacy of extended-release inject-able naltrexone (XR-naltrexone) compared to placebo was determined by Russian studies; the FDA based its approval for OUD on these studies as well as on the safety profile established for XR-naltrexone in the treat-ment of alcohol use disorder. More recent studies raise concerns about the efficacy of XR-naltrexone compared with methadone or buprenorphine in important outcome measures for opioid use disorder (e.g., overdose preven-tion; Wakeman et al., 2020).

ONGOING HEALTH STATUS MONITORING AND TESTING

While in treatment, toxicology testing is typically left to the discretion of the treating clinician, unless it is embedded in regulations associated with the treatment, such as in OTPs where methadone is dispensed, or when treatment is mandated by a criminal justice agreement. When left to clini-cal judgment, toxicology testing may be done infrequently if patients are assessed as doing well. People not in treatment generally do not participate in toxicology testing unless involved in a monitoring program, most typi-cally through their work or the criminal justice system.

Jarvis and colleagues (2017) made a number of recommendations in an ASAM consensus statement titled *Appropriate Use of Drug Testing in Clinical Addiction Medicine*, including that testing should be more frequent during the beginning of treatment and decreased depending on progress. Additionally, testing should be done at least monthly "when a patient is stable in treatment," and that "individual consideration may be given for less frequent testing if a patient is in stable recovery" (Jarvis et al., 2017).

For safety-sensitive professionals, with abstinence viewed as a critical outcome, biologic measures are especially prominent in monitoring health status to prevent impairment at work. Although substance use may not in itself suffice to define relapse into an active disease state, agreements that allow safety-sensitive professionals to return to work are typically clear that substance use could and usually will result in removal from work. This is not to say that clinical judgment of treatment engagement and response from clinicians providing treatment to safety-sensitive pro-fessionals are unimportant, or that perceptions from the worksite are unimportant in assessing a professional's health. Rather, clinical and worksite monitors may not be sufficiently sensitive to relapse, particularly if it begins in a limited way. In contrast, random testing provides an objec-tive measure of substance use when indicated and sufficiently frequent, using a variety of testing matrices (Jarvis et al., 2017).

A variety of testing matrices have been developed to detect substance use, each with benefits and limitations. Urine is the most common matrix used. Breath alcohol content can also provide concentrations of alcohol use and provide critical information if levels correlate with impairment. In a monitoring program that expects alcohol abstinence, breath alcohol with its relatively narrow window of detection may need to be supplemented with urine or blood alcohol metabolite testing. A variety of at-home breathalyzer and urine drug testing options are now available to support long-term sobriety (e.g., BACtrack, RecoveryTrek, PROOF Testing, Soberlink). These tests provide observation through cellular devices, commonly in the form of photo or video at the time of sample, making regular testing more convenient and available over weekends and holidays.

Outcomes for physicians in structured monitoring programs—in which a positive test will reliably result in being removed from work—are reported to be the best in addiction treatment. It is possible that toxicology monitoring with clear contingencies for positive tests is an important driver of these reported outcomes, but there is almost no research on whether toxicology testing, as opposed to other aspects of treatment, improves treatment outcomes (Jarvis et al., 2017). Consensus opinion, however, recommends the use of toxicology testing in assessment and monitoring to support recovery (Jarvis et al., 2017).

SPECIAL CONSIDERATIONS ACROSS THE SPECTRUM OF TREATMENT OF SUBSTANCE USE DISORDERS FOR PROFESSIONALS IN SAFETY-SENSITIVE OCCUPATIONS

Well-regarded guidelines for best practices, such as ASAM's, that are built on "a foundation of evidence… and expert consensus" (American Society of Addiction Medicine, n.d.),[8] assert that due to the concerns for public safety when a professional in a safety-sensitive occupation has a substance use disorder, "treatment should be aggressive and definitive" (Mee-Lee et al., 2013). ASAM therefore recommends that professionals in safety-sensitive occupations participate in treatment that "has the best chance of establishing stable recovery." This approach to identifying the appropriate level of care is notably different from what is recommended for the general population. It is not clear from research which treatment elements of what is proposed as "aggressive and definitive" produce benefits. Individualized treatment combined with accountability through rigorous monitoring and MHGs produces positive effects, yet any one of these elements alone may not be sufficient. However, across treatment programs there are best practices and recommended elements that have emerged that are particularly relevant to the success of treating professionals in

---

[8]For more information on the ASAM Criteria evidence base, see https://www.asam.org/asam-criteria/about-the-asam-criteria/evidence-base

safety-sensitive occupations such as pilots and flight attendants. The key elements the committee selected for consideration include individualized care and required length of stay, role of stigma, use of MAT, release of information and confidentiality, and having access to a cohort of peers. Each is discussed next, in turn.

Individualized Care and Required Length of Stay

While duration of treatment, sometimes referred to as length of stay (LOS), should be individualized based on ongoing assessments using the ASAM dimensions, a recommended level of care and LOS are often assumed for pilots because of the high risk to the public in the event of a relapse. HIMS most commonly expect pilots who meet the FAA definition of substance abuse and dependence to engage in residential treatment, regardless of severity of substance use disorder, and to have a minimum LOS at this level of care of roughly 30 days. This requirement of residential treatment is consistent with what is typically required of physicians with substance use disorders involved in physician health programs; their LOS in residential care most commonly ranges from 30 to 90 days (McLellan et al., 2008). For many professionals who do not seek treatment until required because of problems at work, their substance use disorder may have progressed to being severe and may necessitate residential treatment. However, in cases of professionals with mild substance use disorders, residential treatment may not be indicated (Boyd & Knight, 2012; DuPont et al., 2009). For example, a physician with an isolated arrest for DUI may not meet criteria for having a substance use disorder nor require treatment at the residential level.

However, research does not clearly indicate that residential treatment is superior to less costly and less confining outpatient levels of care (Beaulieu et al., 2021; McCarty et al., 2014). Depending on the structure, a residential program might not offer more intensive treatment than an outpatient program nor meet the unique needs of the individual requiring treatment. Residential treatment is often cited as contributing to good outcomes for professionals in safety-sensitive occupations, yet it is unclear from research whether this is as important as ongoing treatment, regular toxicology monitoring, engagement in a professional monitoring program, or the combination of these elements (Beauliu et al., 2021; McCarty et al., 2014). Moreover, many professionals in safety-sensitive occupations do not complete these lengthy residential stays yet are able to obtain recovery, both people known to their professional monitoring organization and those seeking care outside of that organization (Beauliu et al., 2021, McCarty et al., 2014). In the clinical experience of some committee members, the requirement of completing residential treatment often checks a box for many professionals; however, poor-quality programs do not provide adequate intervention, do not individualize the care, and often let the professional dictate their care in ways that are problematic. Individual PHP, HIMS, and FADAP identify which treatment providers are acceptable for their participants; however, these lists are always evolving and are typically not public, and the criteria used for identifying acceptable treatment programs are unknown.

Another challenge of residential treatment is that it is expensive. Very few insurance plans will cover a 30- to 90-day residential LOS that pilots and physicians are held to. Many professionals go into significant debt to successfully complete treatment, maintain compliance with their professional monitoring organization, and return to work; this financial burden then becomes a clinical issue for many.[9] For example, a survey of 133 physicians who had completed a PHP monitoring agreement for their substance use disorder at least five years in the past (by January 2009) found that out-of-pocket personal costs ranged from \$250 to \$321,000 (M = \$31,528, SD = \$39,570; Merlo et al., 2022). A further challenge potentially facing pilots is gaining admission and clearance from insurance to get into required residential treatment when a pilot meets the FAA definition of abuse or dependence but does not meet the DSM-5 definition of a substance use disorder. People who cannot pay may be discharged before successfully completing the clinically recommended treatment, which can result in a discharge against clinical advice, complicating the pilot or physician's return to work.

In the clinical experience of some committee members, few safety-sensitive professionals are required to comply with clinical recommendations of 30 to 90 days in residential treatment, most commonly physicians and pilots. Other safety-sensitive professionals, including flight attendants, nurses, train engineers, law enforcement, and attorneys, typically engage in residential treatment as dictated by insurance coverage.

Stigma and Fear of Job Loss

The public often holds stigmatized views toward individuals with mental illness, and the intensity of these stigmatized views is greater for substance use disorders than for other psychiatric disorders (Yang et al., 2017). The experience of stigma itself is associated with an increased risk for substance use (National Academies of Sciences, Engineering, and Medicine, 2016) and considered a social determinant of health. Experiences of stigma can be distinctive, depending on the context. For example,

---

[9]Information from a committee-hosted public workshop, available https://www.nationalacademies.org/event/11-01-2022/workshop-on-dealing-with-substance-use-disordersand-strengthening-well-being-in-commercial-aviation

individuals with opioid use disorders can experience greater stigma than people who use alcohol because, unlike alcohol, some opioids are used illicitly (Kennedy-Hendricks et al., 2017). The experience of stigma can arise from structural, public or social, and internalized sources. These different categories of stigma intersect with other factors such as race, gender, socioeconomic status, age, professional identity, and sexual orientation, potentially contributing to challenges in seeking or obtaining treatment (Cheetham et al., 2022; see Box 3-3).

The stigma of having a substance use disorder remains pervasive in our culture, and it is further heightened for professionals in safety-sensitive occupation (Roche et al., 2019). This stigma is exacerbated by professions that come with prestige and work environments that expect their employees to perform at optimal levels despite significant strains. Thus, when a professional is required to seek a substance use assessment, they are motivated to keep their career and may attempt to delay or avoid treatment as a result. The image of being a professional conflicts with what people have internalized as being *an addict*, preventing them from recognizing they need help and seeking the support. In the committee's professional experience, this stigma facilitates the progression of the disease. Additionally compounding this, racial and ethnic minority groups more often experience mental health stigma (Eylem et al., 2020); this perhaps suggests that pilots working among white-majority colleagues who identify as a person of color or as a member of a marginalized community might need additional supports as part of the prevention and treatment of their substance use disorder.

Stigma is integrated and reinforced through workplace policies, insurance coverage, and support made available to employees if they report a problem, their work suffers as a result of a problem, or they are identified as being under the influence at work. As an example, the FAA requires the disclosure of all care sought on the Application for Medical Certification (FAA Form 8500-8); this form is completed by commercial pilots every 6 to 12 months. HIMS and the FAA are public in their support for and encouragement of pilots seeking help and report that it is a myth that substance use treatment is not allowed. The dilemma is that pilots could interpret some questions on that application form as being in direct conflict with HIMS' and the FAA's statement. For example, one question requires pilots to report all visits to health professionals within the last three years, including the date, name, address, type of health professional, and the reason for the visit. Pilots lie on this form if they do not report having sought help or seek help through out-of-pocket resources. While the FAA is duly obliged to monitor pilot health, it could unintentionally cause a public-safety risk if some pilots are avoiding needed care to be in compliance with this rule and maintain the medical certificate needed for their job. One study of pilots in Norway sheds light on underreporting; nearly 12 percent of pilots in this

---

BOX 3-3
Categories of Stigma Toward Individuals with
Substance Use Disorders

Structural

Structural or institutional stigma exists at the systems or macro level and is enacted through rules, policies, and practices that constrain the opportunities and resources of the stigmatized group. Examples include:

- Underfunding treatment for opioid use disorder and inequitable allocation of resources
- Systemic separation of substance use treatments from physical and mental health services, and
- Policies that create barriers to accessing evidence-based treatments (e.g., requiring a waiver to prescribe medication-assisted treatment).

Public/Social

Public stigma refers to stereotypes and negative attitudes that result in prejudice and discrimination. Examples include:

- Negative core beliefs in society about substance use disorders and treatment (e.g., "addicts are typically homeless people")
- Social hesitancy to supply and expand naloxone in mainstream health, and
- Fear of bad influence arising from community support for harm reduction efforts, such as safe consumption facilities, thinking that such efforts would encourage drug use.

Internalized

Internalized stigma denotes negative thoughts and feelings that arise from identification with a stigmatized group. Examples include:

- Reinforcing a low sense of entitlement to quality care
- Delay in seeking treatment to avoid being "labeled" (e.g., pilots can't have substance use problems), and
- Increased engagement in risky behavior such as needle sharing or avoiding syringe exchanges.

SOURCE: Data from Cheetham et al., 2022.

---

study (N = 1,616) admitted to underreporting information to their AME about one or more conditions, some even acknowledging that their underreporting may have affected flight safety "some" or to a "high extent." The number of pilots underreporting was higher for commercial pilots (nearly 16%) in comparison to other medical classes (Strand et al., 2022) and

5.5 percent of participants underreported related to their drug and alcohol use. Furthermore, 49 percent of responders reported knowing a colleague who had underreported information, and 31 percent believed this affected flight safety "to a high extent" (Strand et al., 2022). Notably, the authors state that "the magnitude of underreporting that is evident in these results just represent a minimum share of the actual magnitude" (Strand et al., 2022, p. 382).

This is also reflected in the rate of reported depression in pilots, which is estimated to be 50 percent higher than the rate among the general population (12.6%) and in the fact that 4.1 percent of commercial pilots report suicidal thoughts (Wu et al., 2016). "The mental well-being of a pilot is paramount to his/her flight safety" (Lewis et al., 2014), yet some pilots could perceive current policies as prohibitive to obtaining mental health care.

While aircraft-assisted pilot suicides are very rare (0.29% of all in-flight fatalities; 8 of 2,758 fatal aviation accidents), all eight airmen involved in clearly documented incidents of this type of suicide between 2003 and 2012 had been medically certified to fly and none had reported mental illness, use of an antidepressant medication, or prior suicide attempts (Lewis et al., 2014). Half of them had disqualifying substances including alcohol, benzodiazepines, and antidepressant medications in their system at the time of the suicide; the two taking antidepressants had not disclosed this to their AME, and no pilot had alerted their AME about depression or suicidal ideation (Lewis et al., 2014).

A study conducted by the National Transportation Safety Board in 2020 indicated that substance use continues to increase among fatally injured pilots (N = 1,042), with the overwhelming majority of incidents occurring in noncommercial, recreational aviation; 28 percent of these pilots between 2013 and 2017 tested positive for at least one substance with the potential to produce impairment, including 48 percent of such pilots in 2017 (National Transportation Safety Board, 2020). The most commonly identified drug was diphenhydramine (Benadryl), an over-the-counter sedating antihistamine. A subset of pilots were identified as using medications that could indicate an underlying impairing condition. For these pilots, the three most common identified drugs were hydrocodone, a sedating opioid used to treat severe pain; citalopram, an antidepressant; and diazepam, a sedating benzodiazepine used to treat severe anxiety and muscle spasms (National Transportation Safety Board, 2020).[10] While the FAA is clear in its stance on the use of impairing substances, a percentage of pilots are using them, obtaining prescriptions, and not reporting these to their AMEs and risking public safety (Strand et al., 2022).

---

[10]After a prepublication version of the report was provided to the FAA, this section was edited to clarify the identified substances with the potential to produce impairment.

The mental well-being of a pilot is paramount to his or her flight safety, yet current policies are perceived as a barrier to seeking mental health care. Decreasing stigma associated with substance use disorder within professional organizations can be an important first step to prevention of disease, including early access to help for professionals in safety-sensitive occupations.

Pilots and Medication for Addiction Treatment

The benefits of any medical treatment must be weighed against the risks posed by treatment, and for professionals in safety-sensitive occupations the risks may be greater given the potential for untoward neurocognitive and motor effects. Current scientific consensus would not support a blanket ban on MATs, as impairment occurs along a range (Kay & Belanger, 2023); instead, each MAT-pilot combination should be context-specific and carefully considered by the AME, consistent with the FAA's policies towards other potentially impairing diagnoses. The Risk Evaluation and Mitigation Strategy is a drug safety program that the FDA can require for medications with serious safety concerns; the Risk Evaluation and Mitigation Strategy helps ensure that the benefits of a medication outweigh its risks. The question should be whether the FAA and other oversight organizations for pilots, flight attendants, and other professionals in safety-sensitive occupations are able to sufficiently evaluate and mitigate the risk associated with MAT.

The majority of flight attendants and pilots with substance use disorders have an alcohol use disorder (HIMS & FADAP, 2022). Some FDA-approved medications for the treatment of alcohol use disorders have few, if any, problematic neurocognitive effects, and motor effects are typically transitory and disappear during treatment (Kay & Belanger, 2023). While these studies do not include pilots (likely for the inherent dangers of conducting a double-blind study on safety-sensitive professionals), a pilot with a substance use disorder could be stabilized using MATs that are deemed likely to be minimally impairing based on the current available science and then tested by the neuropsychologist. If impairment is present, they could be taken off the medication and re-evaluated.

Fewer pilots in HIMS have opioid-related difficulties and opioid use disorders; however, the relapse rate to opioids in the HIMS program is higher than that for alcohol use disorders. These numbers, if they match national trends, may be on the rise, and the number of flight attendants with opioid-related difficulties and opioid use disorders may be higher than that of pilots. Rates of opioid use disorder have been trending upward for decades, and kratom is becoming more widely used; it activates the opioid receptors, and it is legal, believed by many to not be addictive, and rarely tested for in standardized drug screens (Olsen et al., 2019).

Some FDA-approved medications for the treatment of opioid use disorders have potential neurocognitive effects (Kay & Belanger, 2023). However, pilots in HIMS are required to complete rigorous neurocognitive assessment and an assessment of relevant motor skills prior to being cleared to return to flying. Thus, pilots stabilized on MAT could be tested and any concerning cognitive impacts would be identified, as in the process described for alcohol use disorder. Both examples would rely heavily on an effective cognitive screen, and it is unclear how much research, if any, has been done by HIMS-trained neuropsychologists to specially look for MAT-related impairment. Given that pilots are often out of work for up to a year in these scenarios, cognitive testing with two to three months of sobriety and stabilization on these medications could still allow time for retesting without the medication if cognitive concerns are present at the time of initial testing.

The FAA's limitations on MAT are overly restrictive by a benefit-to-risk analysis based on the best available evidence as previously described.[11] Professionals in safety-sensitive occupations would benefit from being offered and encouraged to use these medications, particularly naltrexone and buprenorphine, to aid their recovery and prevent relapse and overdose, both during withdrawal management and as ongoing treatment. Providing the most powerful intervention for treating opioid use disorders would significantly decrease the rate of relapse and minimize the risk of overdose for pilots, flight attendants, and other professionals in safety-sensitive occupations.

ROIs and Confidentiality

ROIs facilitate communication among treatment providers, programs, collateral contacts, identified supports, and professional monitoring organizations. Without ROIs, patients can maintain complete confidentiality over their treatment involvement, sometimes to their detriment due to minimization as noted above and lack of collateral information. Many professional monitoring organizations, including HIMS (but not FADAP), require an open ROI, which must allow for any and all information and records to be provided by the treatment provider. Not having such an ROI on file can result in the participant being out of compliance with their monitoring agreement, which in turn can lead to the professional being out of work longer and being reported to their licensing board. While there is a valid public safety reason to differentiate, HIMS requires that the full treatment record be included in records reviewed by the AME during their

---

[11]After a prepublication version of the report was provided to the FAA, this section was edited to accurately reflect FAA policies.

consideration of a pilot's return to the cockpit, whereas flight attendants have complete confidentiality through FADAP.

The resulting dilemma (with no easy resolution) is that for many patients in safety-sensitive occupations involved with oversight organizations, this ROI is seen as a barrier to full disclosure in treatment. When the monitoring program is not seen as supportive, people are more likely to withhold information out of fear of the consequences for their career (Strand et al., 2002). These patients often withhold trauma histories and minimize mental health symptoms out of fear that their oversight organization will have these details and prevent them from returning to work. This underreporting prevents the patient from receiving the care they truly need, and for many it can lead to requiring repeat episodes of treatment. This issue intersects with the importance of individualizing treatment and the concern for public safety. Treatment plans for people experiencing symptoms related to trauma must take this into consideration; it changes treatment goals and recommendations made. Not addressing symptoms of anxiety and depression can disrupt the functionality of the coping skills taught.

It is well documented that co-occurring disorders complicate the course of recovery; however, recovery is possible if these issues are addressed concurrently with the substance use disorder. While communication with professional monitoring organizations is important, limited ROIs could facilitate this while providing increased confidentiality to the patient. Working with treatment providers or centers that have a thorough understanding of the unique needs of professionals in safety-sensitive occupations and the needs of their monitoring organizations can ensure that both the patients' and the oversight organizations' needs are met.

A full medical record review by a monitoring organization is not necessary for a safe return to work for most professionals in safety-sensitive occupations. A review of the patient discharge summary—including diagnoses, general course of treatment progress, clinical recommendations, discharge plan, and recovery support—may be sufficient for review, particularly if the monitoring program receives updates throughout treatment. While the full record has to be released for pilots, it is unlikely that the full record, including every group, individual, and milieu therapy note, is actually being reviewed. The dilemma is that, while ROIs can facilitate communication among providers and professional monitoring organizations, an ROI that requires the release of the full medical record may be a barrier to necessary disclosures in treatment and can infringe on pilots receiving the care they need to maintain public safety.

Peers in Recovery

It is recommended by ASAM and supported by professional monitoring programs that professionals in safety-sensitive occupations benefit greatly from group therapy with peers in similar professions. While literature on this topic is lacking, ASAM reflects "a foundation of evidence around the multidimensional factors that influence disease severity and prognosis and expert consensus from a broad coalition of clinical stakeholders" (American Society of Addiction Medicine, n.d.). Peers in such a cohort help normalize conversations about the impact addiction has had professionally and how the disease has put others at risk and challenged public trust in the profession. Additionally, within a group of peers individuals can more easily hold each other accountable in staying sober, as professional status does not inherently elevate one over another. Professional peers can also challenge each other constructively due to their similar ways of thinking about the world and their understanding of the profession. Conversely, both peers and untrained clinical staff who are unfamiliar with the professional identity often let risky behaviors slide because they look up to these professionals, do not understand their needs, want to be liked by them, or experience countertransference. A significant level of privilege comes with the status of being a safety-sensitive professional; this privilege can lead to excessive self-reliance and difficulty asking for help and taking on the necessary role of being a patient.

Selecting a Treatment Program

Professional monitoring organizations dictate which treatment programs are acceptable for care. Airline HIMS and FADAP identify which programs are acceptable for their pilots and flight attendants; however, the criteria used for selecting programs are unclear and options are not always provided. While it is important that treatment programs have expertise in meeting the unique needs of these professionals, the patient should be given options among approved programs and allowed to choose between them. This is a client-centered practice that can improve efficacy of treatment. Potential conflicts of interest arise when an organization allows their employees to attend only one treatment program: this exacerbates concerns of confidentiality for the professional needing treatment and reinforces the belief that the treatment center works for or too closely with the monitoring organization. In general, the criteria that airlines are using to select and approve treatment programs or providers are unclear, and a range of treatment options is not always provided, which can reduce the likelihood of treatment effectiveness.

Psychological Testing as Part of Treatment

Treatment programs working with this population must understand when it is appropriate and when it is necessary to incorporate psychological testing. Beyond understanding the general appropriateness and benefit to patient care that psychological testing offers, integrating psychological testing may be necessary for some professionals and problematic for others. For example, psychological testing of pilots should be completed by HIMS-trained and board-certified neuropsychologists. Testing by treatment providers can interfere with these evaluations; psychologists delivering testing as part of treatment need to be aware of which measures they can use without interfering with the mandated testing through the neuropsychologist for return-to-duty evaluations with pilots. While psychological testing could be beneficial in making determinations for fitness for duty for all professionals in safety-sensitive occupations, flight attendants and other transportation professionals are not required to complete this type of assessment. Their LOS in treatment is also typically shorter and prohibitive of obtaining a true, current baseline understanding of cognitive functioning; sober time is needed to obtain this.

Discharge Planning

Treatment providers must understand the unique challenges for return to work as part of discharge planning for professionals in safety-sensitive occupations. As noted above, people with substance use disorders will benefit from engaging in a continuum of addiction care, stepping down through the levels of care to increase their chances for long-term recovery and stepping up as needed. This is not a luxury afforded to all professionals in safety-sensitive professions and can be prohibited by cost of care and availability of time off for treatment.

As an example, pilots who are identified as needing treatment are typically grounded for up to a year, and many airlines ensure the required 28–30 days of treatment are covered by their insurance plans. The time away from work would facilitate a gradual step-down through the continuum of addiction care. The pilot's position is most commonly held until the pilot can safely return to the cockpit. Many pilots complete 30 days of treatment and then step down to aftercare (e.g., meetings with their AME, Birds of a Feather meetings, sometimes outpatient treatment). This built-in structure of not returning to work for an extended period of time affords pilots the opportunity to participate in a more gradual step-down through the levels of care without feeling pressure to return to work. Flight attendants, however, are typically dependent on treatment that can be covered by their insurance. Some airline FADAP have negotiated with their insurance plans to cover 28–30 days in a FADAP-approved treatment program. This agreement ensures that the treatment program is regularly receiving referrals and that the flight attendant is getting the dictated days of treatment; however, the flight attendant typically returns to work immediately following this treatment episode.

Given how their work schedules are made, flight attendants can rarely participate in a gradual step-down through the continuum of care. Instead, they regularly go directly from one of the highest levels of addiction treatment back to a routine work environment with long and irregular hours, access to alcohol, and minimal oversight and accountability. Structured time and consistency are typically encouraged for early recovery, but this is not an option for flight attendants. Furthermore, their salaries are significantly lower than those of pilots, and their health benefits are usually less comprehensive; thus, time away from work is less feasible (Bureau of Labor Statistics, 2022b, 2023). Flight attendants are also more likely to be let go when a substance use problem is discovered; they are regarded as replaceable whereas pilots are more highly valued given the extensive training required to obtain that position.[12] Airlines are more willing to invest in their most highly specialized and highly paid employees, and insurance benefits and medical leave often vary by position. Thus, professionals in different safety-sensitive professions get different access to care and support, even within the same company; while this may be financially practical, these company policies do not align with best practices for obtaining and sustaining long-term recovery or for minimizing risks of burnout and encouraging mental health.

Leveraging MHGs in Recovery

MHGs, also known as self-help groups, are groups of two or more people who share an experience or problem and who come together to provide problem-specific help and support to one another (Humphreys, 2004). Members themselves run groups in rented venues, without professional involvement. And, unlike professional interventions, people can attend MHGs as intensively and for as long as they desire, without the use of insurance, without cost, and without having to divulge personally identifying information. In contrast to professional treatment, people typically have access to MHGs at times when they are at higher risk of relapse, such as evenings and weekends, and many MHGs encourage members to contact each other by telephone between meetings whenever help is needed. Consequently, these organizations provide an adaptive, community-based system that is highly responsive to undulating relapse risk (Kelly & Yeterian, 2011).

---

[12]FADAP staff response to the committee-issued questionnaire, August 2022.

Many MHGs exist for people with substance use disorders, including Alcoholics Anonymous (AA), Cocaine Anonymous, Narcotics Anonymous (NA), SMART Recovery, Recovery Dharma, Birds of a Feather, and Wings of Sobriety. AA has been the most researched, however. The benefits of AA for alcohol-related problems have been identified in a meta-analysis published in 2009 (Kaskutas, 2009) where abstinence was an important measure.[13] Aspects of AA that have been demonstrated to mediate its success include identification and connection with other members of the fellowship (e.g., through sponsorship) and involvement in work that contributes to the ability of the organization to help others with problems with alcohol ("service work"). There is less evidence for the effectiveness of NA than there is for AA, but one study finds that retention and benefit for individuals with non-alcohol substance use disorders are comparable whether such individuals join AA or NA (Kelly et al., 2014). Many people sustain recovery through participation in other mutual support groups as well, including SMART Recovery, Dharma Recovery, and more community-specific options tied to their personal interests (e.g., music, fitness) and identities (e.g., MHGs for LGBTQ+ people, for women, for dads).

AA is often described as featuring "treatment" and "self-help." However, AA meetings are not led or guided by addiction treatment professionals, although on-site AA meetings are often embedded as part of treatment programs. Rather than being purely self-help, AA provides mutual help and peer support. Participation in AA is voluntary; newer members are often escorted by concerned family members, friends, treatment programs, and AA sponsors. Court decisions have ruled against mandatory AA involvement, arguing that the religious and/or spiritual tone of the language of AA violates the rights of those who are nonreligious (e.g., God is referenced in Steps 3, 5, 6, 7, and 11). There is evidence that other mutual help approaches are as effective as AA (Kelly et al., 2020). In keeping with this, court decisions have not ruled against requiring mutual help involvement, but they have ruled against requiring AA when other mutual help options are available.

In the committee's professional experience, while there are benefits of voluntary involvement in fellowship support, participants report that it is the social connections with people who support abstinence, participation in service work, and increased confidence in the ability to maintain sobriety in social situations that are most strongly connected with recovery success. These benefits can be obtained from mutual support groups beyond AA, yet HIMS and FADAP strongly encourage their participants to engage in

---

[13]See also the conclusions of a 2020 Cochrane review on AA and 12-step facilitation programs, https://www.cochrane.org/news/new-cochrane-review-finds-alcoholics-anonymous-and-12-step-facilitation-programs-help-people

AA and the AA-based profession-specific groups, Birds of a Feather[14] for pilots and Wings of Sobriety for flight attendants.

The religious overtones that are part of most AA groups often dissuade spiritually diverse people from participation. However, many people who do not identify as religious have found benefit from these MHGs if they can overcome the religious connotation and connect with the spiritual principles and a higher power of their choosing. The FAA cannot mandate AA due to its reference to God, and requiring AA as a condition of employment would likely violate Title VII of the Civil Rights Act of 1964, which protects employees against discrimination on the basis of religion (or lack thereof). Nevertheless, the HIMS highly recommends AA for most of its participants.[15]

---

[14]Birds of a Feather was formed in response to the need for meeting places for pilots and cockpit crewmembers related to recovery from alcoholism, and is not tied to any company, government institution, or treatment center. It is, however, based on AA. For more on Birds of a Feather, see https://www.boaf.org/

[15]See *EEOC v. United Airlines Inc.*, Civil Action No. 20-cv-9110 (https://www.eeoc.gov/newsroom/united-airlines-pay-305000-settle-eeoc-religious-discrimination-lawsuit). See also several similar First Amendment cases, e.g., *Inouye v. Kemna*, 504 F.3d 705 (9th Cir. 2007); *Warner v. Orange County Dept. of Probation*, 173 F.3d 120 (2d Cir. 1999); *Griffin v. Coughlin*, 88 N.Y. 2d 674 (N.Y. App. Ct. 1996); *Kerr v. Farrey*, 95 F.3d 472 (7th Cir. 1996); *Warburton v. Underwood*, 2 F. Supp. 2d 306 (W.D. N.Y. 1998); *Arnold v. Tennessee Bd. of Paroles*, 956 S.W.2d 478 (Tenn. 1997).

4

A Program Evaluation Overview for Support of Pilots and Flight Attendants with Substance Use Disorders

Pilots and flight attendants operate in a stressful environment that is shaped by public policies and expectations for accountability. This chapter illuminates the larger context in which pilots and flight attendants work, with the goal of describing how evaluation could be employed to better understand whether current supports are adequate for addressing substance use disorders and ensuring their well-being. For this purpose, the chapter first provides a framework that outlines the multiple influences on the work of pilots and flight attendants and includes public policies, airline policies and cultures, workplace stressors, and individual factors. Next, it draws upon the findings laid out in Chapter 3 on the key elements of evidence-based practices for identification and treatment of substance use disorders, and then reviews best practices in program evaluation, to propose key elements to include in evaluations of substance use disorder programs. Finally, evaluation tools used by the Human Intervention Motivational Study (HIMS) and the Flight Attendant Drug and Alcohol Program (FADAP) are discussed in light of how well these align with best practices for program monitoring and assessment. This is followed by recommendations for ways the Federal Aviation Administration (FAA) can improve oversight of substance use disorder programming.

Many stressors can affect the performance of both pilots and flight attendants, but the legally required testing and subsequent severe penalties for alcohol and drug use placed on pilots in particular impose even more stress on pilots, some of whom may be struggling with personal issues that result in their coping through substance use.

85

FACTORS THAT FACILITATE OR IMPEDE PILOTS AND FLIGHT ATTENDANTS FROM SEEKING TREATMENT WHEN NEEDED

This section reviews four types of factors that may facilitate or impede pilots' and flight attendants' willingness to seek treatment when needed. As shown in Figures 4-1 and 4-2, the four types include input factors, external factors, individual factors, and organizational factors that lead to desired outcomes of capable pilots, flight attendants, and airline safety.

Inputs

Input factors are those that may influence an employee's decision to pursue substance use disorder treatment. These include pilot/flight attendant characteristics, public accountability, and policies at various levels that may dictate or influence behavior. Pilot-related characteristics may impact whether and how they seek treatment when they have substance use disorders. DeHoff and Cusick (2018) also point out that the distinctive nature of the occupation of pilots may also impact their willingness to seek help when they have depression, anxiety, and other mental illness. Pilots are more prone to hazardous attitudes such as invulnerability and macho (e.g., "It won't happen to me" and "I can do it"; DeHoff & Cusick, 2018), which is likely to prevent them from seeking help when needed.

Public accountability is another significant factor, one that impacts pilots' and flight attendants' tendency to seek medical treatment. The physical and mental health of the pilots and flight attendants is important to the safety of flight, which is critical to the airline, the passengers, and the public. Indeed, flight accidents are usually associated with serious injuries and fatalities, which cause severe loss to the public and cumulative decreases in enplanement for the airlines (Insua et al., 2019 Squalli & Saad, 2006). Therefore, pilots, flight attendants, and airlines share the responsibility to ensure the safety of their flights. The policies of the FAA, unions, and airlines may also influence pilots' and flight attendants' willingness to seek treatment. For example, flight crews may hesitate to seek help due to a concern about the potential impacts on their medical certification process. The *Guide for Aviation Medical Examiners* requires that an employee reporting any mental condition "requires investigation through supplemental history taking," that "dispositions will vary according to the details obtained," (FAA, 2023b), and that this finding be reported to the FAA (DeHoff & Cusick, 2018).[1] Consequently, flight crews' perceived risks of interrupting their careers may be a hurdle for them to seek needed assistance. In addition,

---

[1]After a prepublication version of the report was provided to the FAA, this section was edited to reflect 2023 FAA Guidance.

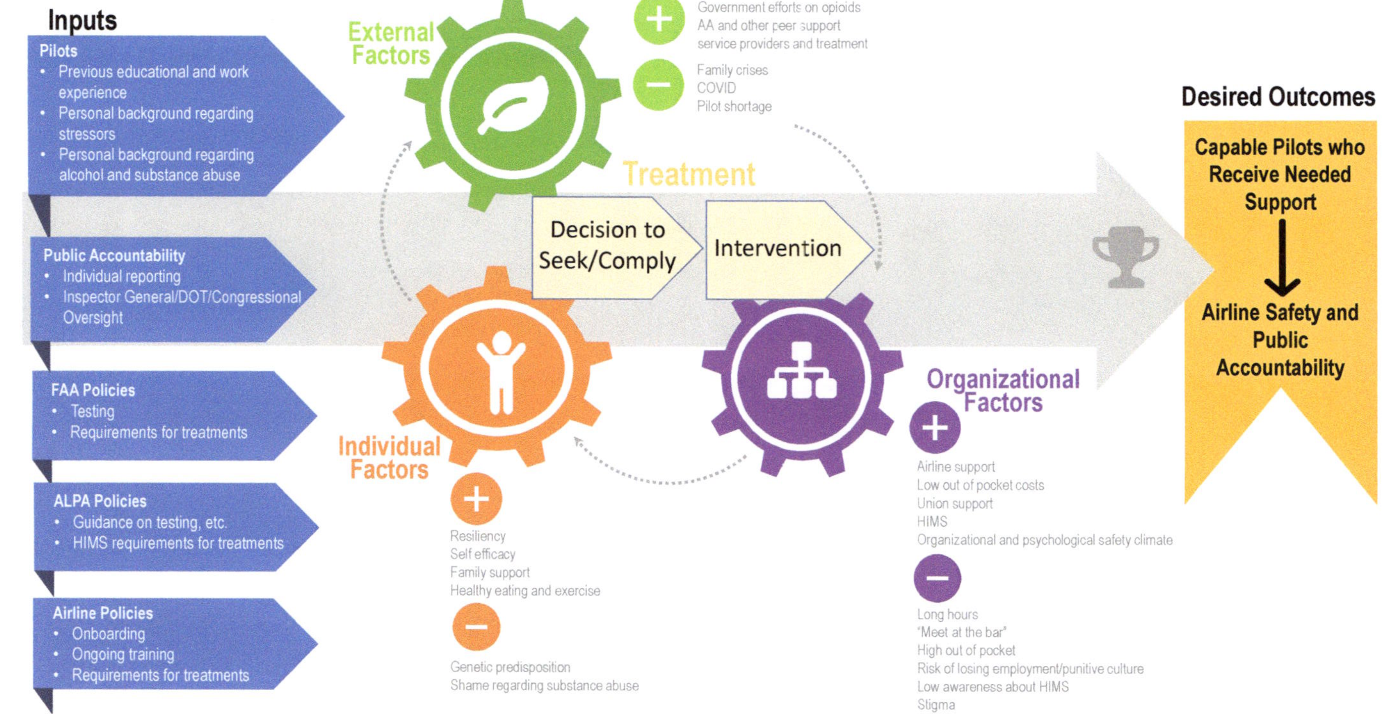

FIGURE 4-1 The context for facilitating pilot well-being and job performance.
NOTE: AA = Alcoholics Anonymous; ALPA = Air Line Pilots Association-International; DOT = U.S. Department of Transportation; FAA = Federal Aviation Administration; HIMS = Human Intervention Motivational Study.

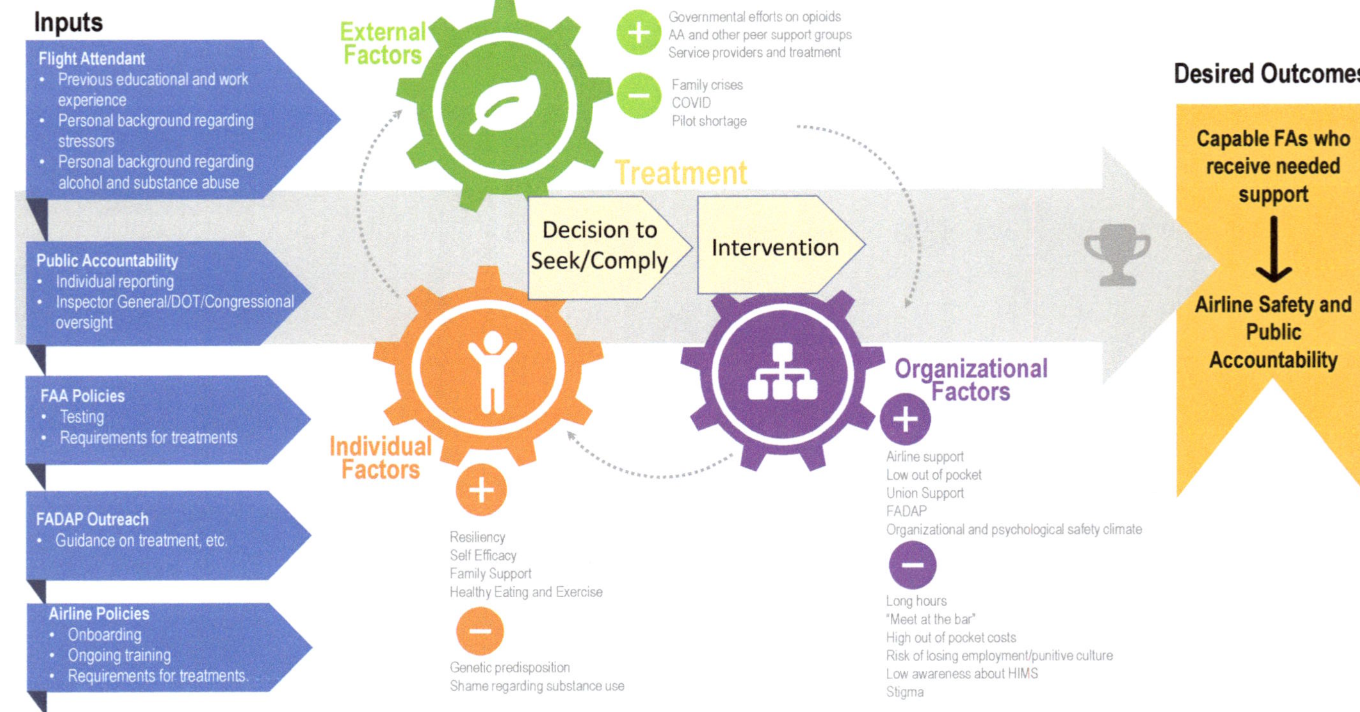

FIGURE 4-2 The context for facilitating flight attendant well-being and job performance.
NOTE: AA = Alcoholics Anonymous; DOT = U.S. Department of Transportation; FA = flight attendant; FAA = Federal Aviation Administration; FADAP = Flight Attendant Drug and Alcohol Program; HIMS = Human Intervention Motivational Study.

airlines' policies may also play a similar role in influencing pilots' and flight attendants' attitudes about seeking treatments. In a study that sampled 221 flight department leaders, 68 percent of respondents indicated that their flight operation had a written substance use policy, but only 20 percent indicated that it had policies on rehabilitation and only 16 percent that it had job retention/recovery policies (Vardiman, 2008). As a result, the flight crews' fear of disrupting their careers may lead to their unwillingness to seek medical treatment when they are involved in substance abuse disorders.

External Factors

Peer support can play a key role in facilitating pilots and flight attendants in obtaining recovery. Alcoholics Anonymous (AA), for example, provides those who have substance use disorders an opportunity to learn about addiction at no cost and from others in a similar situation. It has a low threshold of inclusion, encourages expressions of one's own personal history and challenges, and helps people build intimate social networks (Westermeyer, 2014). AA and other mutual help groups can be especially helpful when involved individuals share similar experiences and characteristics (e.g., Birds of a Feather, Wings of Recovery or similar cultures; Westermeyer, 2014). These groups also help people recognize that while their profession or socioeconomic status may differ from others' in these groups, they have the same disease and have more in common than they initially perceived. Both FADAP and HIMS include peer support as a foundation of their program.

In addition to the social-emotional support from peers, professional support from addiction experts and treatment programs are also important facilitators of flight crews' health and well-being. When pilots or flight attendants have substance use disorders, appropriate medical services and treatments are critical for their recovery (Horton et al., 2010, 2011; Shorey et al., 2014). HIMS and FADAP are designed to connect employees with such treatment.

While many external facilitators can help flight crew members obtain treatment when needed, other external factors may stop them from receiving these treatments and make their situation more stressful. For example, one important factor is related to their family. While supportive families can be key to encouraging help seeking, pilots and flight attendants are prone to having strained family dynamics. Difficulty finding time they can spend with their families during peak work times and missing important family events due to their work responsibilities (Cullen et al., 2021) causes strain. For this reason, their spouses may also suffer due to the inability of pilots and flight attendants to take up their share of domestic or parental roles (Cullen et al., 2021). Additionally, due to the limited usage of cell phones on flights, pilots and flight attendants may also find it hard to participate in school-related activities for their children (Butcher, 2002; Foster & Ren, 2015; Ren & Foster, 2011). All these pressures related to family issues can add to the stress in pilots' and flight attendants' lives and may even intensify their reliance on alcohol or drugs.

Another, more recent, adverse factor that has emerged is COVID-19. Since the outbreak of the global pandemic in early 2020, the economy has inevitably suffered greatly, especially in the travel industry. Some areas were locked down, and others set strict policies about passengers' health status. Consequently, the airlines have experienced significant decreases in revenues. This external shock has led to uncertainty and insecurity for pilots and flight attendants regarding their future careers and their medical certifications (Suthatorn & Charoensukmongkol, 2022; Troyer & Bidaisee, 2022; Xiao et al., 2022), which makes their situation worse, especially for those with substance use disorders.

The projected industrywide pilot shortage may also aggravate pilots' and flight attendants' occupational stressors and prevent them from accessing effective treatment. Klapper and Ruff-Stahl (2019) estimate that regional airlines would face a deficit of about 5,000 to 8,000 pilots by 2023. This may be translated to increased workloads and reduced break time, thereby creating stressors and reduced possibility of getting timely treatments.

Individual Factors

A range of individual factors can also facilitate or impede pilots' and flight attendants' treatment-seeking when they are in need. Resiliency represents an individual's strengths and means of coping with stressors and adversity (Richardson, 2002). Resilient individuals are more likely to successfully handle stressors and deal with disruptions, and thus help themselves heal from the harmful impacts of substance use with the right treatment. Self-efficacy is the belief in one's abilities to produce designated levels of performance and exercise influence over events that affect their lives (Bandura, 1982). Those with higher levels of self-efficacy may believe that they can change their own situations and may thus spend efforts to seek treatments for their own recovery. While research has also shown that self-efficacy is an important predictor of post-treatment abstinence, this can also be a barrier to treatment success for professionals, who can be *too* self-reliant, limiting their willingness to ask for or otherwise seek help (Kadden & Litt, 2011).

Healthy eating and exercise can also help pilots and flight attendants in this situation, just as they have been found to benefit physical and mental health in general. Indeed, healthy eating and exercise can serve as preventive and therapeutic interventions to prevent and treat mental illness and substance use disorders (Zschucke et al., 2012). In addition to the factors related to themselves, factors related to their significant others may also play a role. When pilots and flight attendants receive family support (e.g., financial support, direct care), they are more likely to take action and seek treatments when needed. In fact, family support in the form of economic assistance and direct care has been linked to substance abuse recovery and substance use reduction (Clark, 2001).

Despite these positive factors, some other individual factors may make pilots and flight attendants more prone to substance use disorders or impede their help-seeking (as described in-depth in Chapter 3). Genetic predisposition is a critical individual factor that helps explain the between-person differences in addiction tendency. Research has found that addiction runs in families (Hall et al., 2015). More direct evidence on human DNA has also provided preliminary support for the potential linkage between genes and addiction (Ball, 2008). Shame is another individual factor that may influence pilots' and flight attendants' tendency to receive treatment. Those with substance use disorders commonly have shame and blame themselves for such problems (O'Connor et al., 1994), which may worsen their situations and even stop them from seeking treatment, adding to internalized stigma related to mental health, as discussed more thoroughly in Chapter 3.

Organizational Factors

Several nonregulatory organizational factors may also impact pilots' and flight attendants' willingness to seek treatment when in need. The level of airline support is one of the most important factors, because pilots' and flight attendants' perceived uncertainty about how treatment or medical history impacts their careers has been identified as one of the most important considerations when they have alcohol or other drug-related problems (DeHoff & Cusick, 2018; Vardiman, 2008).

Airline Financial Support

Inadequate financial support from airlines for treatment presents an especially important factor. For example, pilots are required to undergo neuropsychological and psychiatric assessments to assess fitness for duty, as well as assessments of the quality and extent of recovery in preparation for application for Special Issuance authorization. However, these required evaluations are typically not reimbursable by insurance carriers, because the evaluations are geared toward regulatory requirements and not clinical diagnostics. These evaluations are often paid for by larger airlines in accordance with collective bargaining agreements. On the other hand, pilots for smaller carriers and regional airlines may have less financial support for these assessments, which can be extremely costly as discussed in Chapter 2 (see cost estimates by treatment modality).

Similarly, airlines vary greatly in the amount of financial support they provide flight attendants who seek treatment. Unlike pilots, for whom the treatment is typically fully covered, flight attendants may face extremely high out-of-pocket costs for treatment, even up to a large proportion of their annual income. Lower out-of-pocket costs would help both flight attendants and pilots receive appropriate treatments, as financial considerations have an unignorable impact on patients' willingness to receive medical services (Clark, 2001). Flight attendants in general, and pilots at smaller airlines, are clearly at more risk of not seeking treatment due to the heavy financial burden they would face. Although we do not know much about the practices in industries with other transportation modes (e.g., trucking, train, shipping), the recommendation for the employer to cover substance use disorder treatment seems to equally apply to other safety-sensitive positions.

Organizational and Psychological Safety Climate

The climates of organizational safety and psychological safety are also important factors affecting the likelihood that pilots and flight attendants will seek treatment for substance use disorder. Within a psychologically safe climate, pilots and flight attendants are less likely to have perceived uncertainty and job insecurity, which may deter them from seeking treatment (Edmondson, 1999). The Department of Labor has resources and guidance for any organization willing to establish a Recovery-Ready Workplace,[2] and several industries with particularly high-stress and safety-sensitive environments have called for an organizational climate of safety and wellness; these industries include (but are not limited to) physicians and nurses (Baldisseri, 2007; DuPont & Skipper, 2012; Shaw et al., 2004), trucking (Arboleda et al., 2003), and law enforcement (Taylor et al., 2022).

The U.S. Department of Transportation (DOT) has defined safety culture as "The shared values, actions, and behaviors that demonstrate a commitment to safety over competing goals and demands" (Morrow & Coplen, 2017, p. 2). DOT further details the 10 most critical elements of a strong safety culture as these:

1. leadership is clearly committed to safety;
2. open and effective communication exists across the organization;
3. employees feel personally responsible for safety;
4. the organization practices continuous learning;
5. the work environment is safety conscious;

---

[2]https://www.dol.gov/agencies/eta/RRW-hub/Recovery-ready-workplace

6. reporting systems are clearly defined and not used to punish employees;
7. decisions demonstrate that safety is prioritized over competing demands;
8. employees and the organization work to foster mutual trust;
9. the organization responds to safety concerns fairly and consistently; and
10. safety efforts are supported by training and resources.

Similarly, Box 4-1 describes five important aspects of a safety culture.

Union Support

Union support may also affect whether or not pilots and flight attendants seek treatment, because unions may contribute to the improvement of relevant organizational policies for flight crew benefits, such as explicit policies about rehabilitation and job retention. Further, professional programs such as HIMS and FADAP can also help pilots and flight attendants when they are in need. However, while HIMS and FADAP can be helpful, it is likely that some pilots and flight attendants are unaware of the existence of these supporting programs. In fact, anecdotal input received by this committee during the committee meetings suggests that the visibility of both HIMS and FADAP can be bolstered.

BOX 4-1
Five Important Aspects of a Safety Culture

1. *Informed*: The organization collects information about both accidents and incidents and carries out proactive countermeasures.
2. *Reporting*: All employees report their errors or near misses and take part in initiatives to improve safety.
3. *Just*: There is an atmosphere of trust within an organization that encourages and rewards its employees for providing information on errors and incidents, with the confidence of knowing that they will receive fair and just treatment for any mistake they make.
4. *Flexible*: The organization and the people in it are capable of adapting effectively to changing demands.
5. *Learning*: The organization learns from incident reports, safety audits, and other activities, resulting in improved safety.

SOURCE: Wisdom, 2022.

It is worth highlighting key aspects of the work scheduling and environment that also may discourage pilots and flight attendants from seeking treatment. Long work hours may decrease their possibility of seeking (and getting) treatment because work occupies too much of their time, rendering them without the temporal and psychological resources to obtain medical services (Andresen et al., 2007). A "meet-at-the-bar" culture may also make it hard for the flight crew members to avoid alcohol or may even normalize their addiction so they stop seeking treatment (Liu et al., 2015). As noted above and discussed in Chapter 3, a punitive culture or the risk of losing employment may also be harmful to pilots' and flight attendants' health and their willingness to receive treatment (DeHoff & Cusick, 2018). In addition, stigma is also a major factor that prevents the flight crew from treatment and confounds their recovery (Corrigan et al., 2017). Because substance misuse is socially discrediting, those in need may mentally deny the existence of such problems or distance themselves from treatment to avoid being regarded as problematic (Corrigan et al., 2017).

KEY ELEMENTS OF GOOD SUBSTANCE USE DISORDER TREATMENT FOR PILOTS AND FLIGHT ATTENDANTS

HIMS and FADAP play important intermediary roles in helping pilots and flight attendants needing support to deal with substance use disorders find and complete appropriate treatment and reenter their work roles successfully. Not all pilots and flight attendants work with HIMS and FADAP to secure support, but the focus of this study is on how HIMS and FADAP can best serve those who do use their services. Both HIMS and FADAP have criteria to judge the providers to whom they refer pilots and flight attendants.[3] Drawing upon the most up-to-date data to emphasize the best practices for substance use disorder treatment (see Chapter 3 for more details), this section outlines highlights and key takeaways.

As a starting point, a key question to ask is: What will success look like for the individuals and the other stakeholders, including unions, the airlines, and the flying public? (See Figure 4-3.) Success, measured by outcomes, may differ across types of stakeholders. "For [alcohol use disorders], health outcomes can be expanded to include four areas: sustained reductions in [alcohol use disorder] use, improvements in personal health, sustained improvements in functioning (e.g., employment), and sustained

---

[3]For FADAP, this process includes conducting interviews both with the participating flight attendant, their peer mentor, and the treating provider and could include review of the flight attendant's treatment file. Request for corrective action by the treatment program or suspension of referrals until corrective action takes place may be the outcome of the quality assurance process.

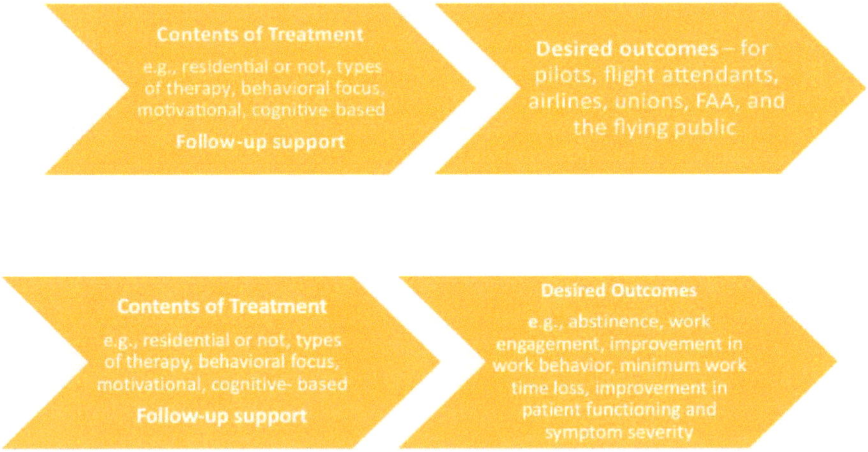

FIGURE 4-3 What makes for an "effective" intervention?

reductions in threats to public health and safety" (Garnick et al., 2006, cited in McLellan et al., 2005). FAA and airline management, for example, may place priority on workplace outcome measures invoking safety in flight operations such as long-term sobriety (abstinence) and rate of return to safety-sensitive duties while program outcomes may focus on treatment effectiveness (rate of relapse) and length of time to enter into treatment from time of identification/referral. From the perspective of individual pilots and flight attendants, success may be spending as little time away from the job as possible. But success in terms of obtaining sobriety and sufficient recovery may take much longer than the individual pilots and flight attendants prefer. Chapter 5 of this report presents statistics on program outcomes, in particular in Tables 5.3 through 5.5. The optimal combination of treatment and recovery support will vary based on the individual needs of a given pilot or flight attendant. There is no standardized treatment plan that will meet all pilot and flight attendant needs, but recognizing that there is not one perfect combination, nor one standard intervention timeline, is a first step.

Continuing care presents an especially important and essential support for pilots and flight attendants with substance use disorders (as described in depth in Chapter 3). It is essential that the recommended continuing care support services be individualized and person-centered, as stated by McKay (2009, p. 12):

There is increasing recognition that many individuals simply do not like some aspects of traditional treatment programs, including the emphasis on total abstinence, pressure to embrace the AA program, reliance on group therapy, and so forth. Conversely, some patients would be willing to attend treatment in specialty care sessions, but are unable to do so because of family responsibilities, transportation problems, and so forth. Therefore, patient preference needs to be taken seriously and not simply seen as indicative of resistance or denial.

Current research does provide guidance on the elements of substance use disorder treatment that have been shown to be effective. A key consideration is what is the most appropriate level of care for entry to treatment. While residential treatment is considered optimal by HIMS and FADAP, as distractions due to family and other demands are reduced, it is often perceived as especially burdensome and overly costly, particularly depending on insurance coverage and financial resources. Many essential elements of good programming for substance abuse disorder treatment were described, based on the available evidence, in Chapter 3. Qualified treatment programs will at least:

- be patient-centered and individualized;
- be guided by American Society of Addiction Medicine standards for assessment and use the biopsychosocial-spiritual model;
- be staffed with professionals holding expertise and advanced clinical credentials;
- offer evidence-based interventions for treating substance use disorders (e.g., appropriately selected and monitored medications, Motivational Interviewing, mindfulness strategies, cognitive behavioral therapy, dialectical behavior therapy, contingency management, and peer support); and
- be trauma-focused and address co-occurring physical and mental health conditions.

EMPLOYING EVALUATION TOOLS

Program evaluation is the application of systematic methods to address questions about program operations and results, and it includes ongoing monitoring of a program as well as one-shot studies of program processes or program impact. Evaluative thinking and use of data collection tools present valuable opportunities for enhancing knowledge about the underlying logic of programs and the program activities under way, as well as about the results of programs (Newcomer et al., 2015). The field of program evaluation offers processes and tools useful for obtaining valid, reliable, and credible data to address a variety of questions about the performance of any program.

A frequently used distinction in evaluation work is between formative and summative evaluation. Formative evaluation uses evaluation methods to improve the way a program is delivered, while summative evaluation entails systematically measuring program outcomes and results during ongoing operations or after program completion. Most evaluation work will examine program implementation to some extent, if only to ensure that the assessment of outcomes or impacts can be logically linked to program activities.

Credible evaluation work requires clear, valid measures that are collected in a reliable, consistent fashion. Evaluation work must begin with clarifying what will constitute credible measures and establishing strong procedures to ensure that both quantitative measurement and qualitative measurement are rigorous. The relevance, legitimacy, and clarity of the data collected on both program implementation and outcomes matter to program stakeholders and the public.

So, how might HIMS and FADAP employ evaluation effectively? Both formative and summative evaluation approaches are needed, as is the collection of valid and reliable data. In particular, data should be collected for the target population (i.e., employees with safety sensitive duties) to determine the effectiveness of prevention efforts as well as the prevalence of substance use disorder (both treated and untreated) in the workplace, in addition to data from all participants (rather than a sample of them) referred to the programs and following treatment completion (see Box 4-2). The research undertaken as part of the committee's work suggests that more careful, complete, and transparent data collection is needed.

In addition to monitoring how well those who complete treatment fare, there are a number of other best practices that both HIMS and FADAP should consider. The committee outlines a set of questions that both programs should address on an ongoing basis to ensure that through their actions they are contributing to the well-being of pilots and flight attendants (see Table 4-1).

BOX 4-2
Key Elements for Good Monitoring and Evaluation
for HIMS and FADAP

Data on Target Population (employees with safety-sensitive duties):
- Percentage of employees (by functional role) who had attended training on the topic of substance use disorder in the workplace
- Rate of awareness on HIMS and FADAP
- Percentage of employees who had received training specific to HIMS and FADAP
- Substance use disorder prevalence and treated substance use disorder in the workplace

Data on All Participants:
- Intake interviews/administrative data
- Preprogram, immediate post-program, and follow-up surveys (6 and 12 months out)
- Data on health status regarding ability to carry out necessary occupational functions

Data on Program:
- How was the treatment customized for patients?
- What was the set of treatments offered to the participant?
- To what extent was treatment learning-oriented? (e.g., offering new tools for self-regulation?)
- What sorts of enrichment tools were offered?

TABLE 4-1 Adherence to Recommended Practices—Considerations for HIMS and FADAP

Questions to Consider
Encouragement for voluntary entry?
Financial support for residential treatment?
Use of appropriate treatment modality?
Individualized treatment and culturally responsive practices?
Clear and justified criteria for selection of treatment programs?
Ongoing sustaining support?
Systematic evaluation of providers?
Continuous monitoring of program effectiveness, cost efficiency, and positive health outcomes?

5

Outcomes of the Human Intervention and Motivational Study and the Flight Attendant Drug and Alcohol Program: Analysis of the Available Evidence

The study committee aimed to ascertain characteristics of the flight attendants and pilots who took part in the Flight Attendant Drug and Alcohol Program (FADAP) and Human Intervention and Motivational Study (HIMS), respectively; the details of their treatment (e.g., length of treatment, whether or not medication-assisted treatment was offered); and measures of program satisfaction and effectiveness. To do this, the committee requested access to the FADAP and HIMS outcome databases for analysis by an independent consultant. In addition, to obtain flight attendants' and pilots' perspectives on the FADAP and HIMS, the committee developed a tool for anonymously gathering experiences (through a "Call for Perspectives") and commissioned a qualitative study involving interviews with flight attendants and pilots. This chapter summarizes the findings from these efforts.

Before presenting the findings, a few comments are warranted. First, the data are characterized by low response rates and/or selection bias, which limit the conclusions we can confidently draw from them. Second, however, this chapter presents these data because it is important to describe what is and is not known. For example, the substantial amount of missing data due to low survey response rates are itself an important finding. Third, much of the data is based on self-reports. Although self-reports can be reliable and valid, they are subject to response biases, such as the social desirability bias—a tendency to answer questions in a way that will be judged favorably by others (Althubaiti, 2016). It is important to be aware of the possibility of under-reporting of substance use. For example, data available to the committee suggest that among both flight attendants and pilots, opioid misuse is relatively infrequent compared to misuse of other substances. It is possible that the available data undercount the actual prevalence of opioid misuse in the aviation industry and continued vigilance related to opioid (mis)use is warranted.

FINDINGS FOR FADAP

Findings from an Independent Analysis of the FADAP Database

FADAP collects data on flight attendant outcomes among those who have received treatment from FADAP-approved residential treatment centers. Flight attendants are asked to complete three surveys:

1. An initial survey administered approximately three weeks into treatment (called "Initial Self-Report Survey," first launched in 2014), which assesses the history of prior treatment, disciplinary actions at work, job performance, treatment engagement, and satisfaction with FADAP;
2. A post-treatment survey administered at three to four weeks after treatment completion (called "Post-treatment Survey," first launched in calendar year 2020), which assesses current employment status and satisfaction with the residential treatment program; and
3. A post-treatment survey administered at one year after treatment completion (called "Follow-up Self-Report Survey," first launched in 2014), which assesses current self-described "recovery" status, current employment status, disciplinary actions at work, current and past job performance, current and past engagement in treatment, and satisfaction with FADAP.

Flight attendants' treatment providers are also asked to complete a survey on each flight attendant's treatment (called "Primary Treatment Summary" survey), which assesses a flight attendant's admission and discharge dates, whether the flight attendant completed the full course of treatment, the flight attendant's presenting problem (e.g., alcohol, drugs, mental health), whether social supports participated in treatment, details of medication-assisted therapy (e.g., whether it was offered, accepted), and the flight attendant's level of engagement in treatment.

The study committee contracted with Cara M. Nordberg (MPH) to conduct an independent analysis of the FADAP database. Key results are briefly summarized here, and the full report can be found in the "Resources" section of this report's website. The data were received in November 2022. The analyzed database comprised data from 1,196 unique flight attendants who were admitted for treatment between June 2014 and October 2022 (with the latest discharge date in November 2022), and 1,172 unique treatment episodes. To be counted as a unique treatment episode by the analyst, treatment providers must have returned the "Primary Treatment Summary" survey with non-missing admission and discharge dates, and repeat treatment episodes had to be separated by at least 28 days.

Completeness of the FADAP Database

Survey response rates are important because they affect interpretation of the findings. When survey response rates are low, findings may be biased because the responses represent only a small subset of the population of interest, and respondents often differ from non-respondents in important ways. For example, prior research has shown that respondents tend to be healthier than nonrespondents (e.g., have less severe substance use and mental health problems), which means that findings based on a small subset of respondents are often biased toward healthier respondents. When survey response rates are high, there is less concern about biased findings, since most of the population (i.e., both severe and non-severe cases) is represented in the data.

Response rates varied across the FADAP surveys. The 1,196 flight attendants showed a fairly high response rate to the "Initial Self-Report Survey" (73.6%, N = 880). Among flight attendants far enough out from treatment and therefore eligible to complete the 3–4 week "Post-treatment Survey" (N = 377) and the one-year "Follow-up Self-Report Survey" (N = 835), response rates were low, at 23.3 percent (N = 88) and 29.6 percent (N = 247), respectively. The low response rate to the "Follow-up Self-Report Survey" administered at one year after treatment is noteworthy, because this is the survey that collects much of the treatment outcome data (e.g., recovery, return to work, post-treatment satisfaction with FADAP). The treatment provider response rate to the "Primary Treatment Summary" survey was high, with treatment summary data available for 82.8 percent (N = 990) of flight attendants.

To ascertain whether there were differences between respondents and nonrespondents, the analyst compared flight attendants and treatment episodes (since flight attendants could have had multiple treatment episodes) that were lost to follow-up versus those that were not. Loss to follow-up was defined as nonresponse to the one-year "Follow-up Self-Report Survey" for flight attendants/treatment episodes at least one year out from treatment (i.e., those who had completed treatment by May 31, 2021). Overall, 797 flight attendants were eligible for the one-year "Follow-up Self-Report Survey," and 69.0 percent (N = 550) of these flight attendants were lost to follow-up (see Table 5-1). Flight attendants who were lost to follow-up did not differ from flight attendants who were not lost to follow-up in terms

TABLE 5-1 A Comparison of Flight Attendants and Treatment Episodes That Were Lost Versus Not Lost to Follow-Up

Characteristic	Flight Attendants (N = 797)[a]		
	Lost to Follow-up (N = 550)	Not Lost to Follow-up (N = 247)	
	N (percent)	N (percent)	P value
Age, mean (standard deviation)	44.2 (11.4)	44.4 (12.0)	.81
Female biological sex	324 (58.0)	142 (57.5)	.71
Completed initial self-report survey	476 (86.6)	225 (91.1)	.068

Characteristic	Treatment Episodes (N = 974)[b]		
	Lost to Follow-up (N = 685)[c]	Not Lost to Follow-up (N = 289)[d]	
	N (%)	N (%)	P value
Treatment-provider-reported broad treatment issue			.37
Alcohol and mental health	329 (50.8)	143 (53.3)	
Alcohol, drugs, and mental health	134 (20.7)	50 (18.7)	
Alcohol only	95 (14.7)	43 (16.0)	
Drugs and mental health	50 (7.8)	11 (4.1)	
Mental health only	17 (2.6)	8 (3.0)	
Alcohol and drugs	16 (2.4)	7 (2.6)	
Drugs only	7 (1.0)	6 (2.2)	
Treatment-provider-reported MATs[e] offered	463 (95.9)	199 (95.7)	.91
Treatment-provider-reported MATs in treatment plan[f]	332 (71.7)	136 (68.3)	.95
Treatment-provider-reported length of treatment, median (IQR[g])	31 (29, 43)	31 (29, 43)	.52
Treatment-provider-reported treatment completion	568 (90.2)	236 (93.3)	.17
Flight-attendant-reported satisfaction with FADAP at the time of the initial survey[h]			
Would recommend FADAP	524 (94.6)	231 (90.9)	.052
Would use FADAP again	519 (93.7)	230 (90.6)	.112
Satisfied with FADAP	499 (90.2)	227 (89.4)	.70
FADAP made it possible to ask for help	495 (89.5)	224 (88.9)	.79
Would not have made it into treatment without FADAP	476 (86.0)	221 (87.0)	.72

NOTES: [a]797 of the 1,196 unique flight attendants in the database were eligible for the one-year "Follow-up Self-Report Survey" based on being discharged from their most recent

treatment episode by May 31, 2021, and lost to follow-up was defined as nonresponse to the one-year follow-up survey among eligible flight attendants. [b]974 of the 1,172 treatment episodes in the database were eligible for the one-year follow-up survey based on discharge dates by May 31, 2021. [c]Due to missing data, Ns ranged from 483 to 648. [d]Due to missing data, Ns ranged from 208 to 268. [e]MATs = medication-assisted treatments. [f]This question was asked only of those who were offered MATs, so the percentages are based on a denominator N of 463 and 199 for the two groups, respectively. [g]IQR = interquartile range. [h]Shows responses of "agree" or "strongly agree."
SOURCE: Data from FADAP database and results from committee's "Call for Perspectives."

of age or biological sex. Flight attendants who were lost to follow-up were slightly, but non-significantly, less likely to have completed the "Initial Self-Report Survey" than flight attendants who were not lost to follow-up (86.6% vs. 91.1%). The analysis of loss to follow-up was limited, in that information was not available about severity of the presenting problem, race, ethnicity, and precise location, all factors shown to affect follow-up in other research (Cleland et al., 2004).

In terms of treatment episodes, 974 episodes were eligible for the one-year "Follow-up Self-Report Survey," and 70.3 percent (N = 685) of these were lost to follow-up (see Table 5-1). Treatment episodes that were lost to follow-up generally did not differ from treatment episodes that were not lost to follow-up in terms of treatment-provider-reported treatment characteristics, offers of medication-assisted treatment, length of treatment, or treatment completion, and flight attendant reports from the "Initial Self-report Survey" (see Table 5-1).

Characteristics of Flight Attendants in FADAP[1]

Table 5-2 shows the characteristics of the 1,196 unique flight attendants who took part in FADAP. Flight attendants were, on average, 44.4 years old (standard deviation = 11.6 years). Most flight attendants were female (57.5%, N = 686), which is unsurprising because the majority of all flight attendants are female. Nearly half of flight attendants were employed by one of two airlines—Airline 1 (25.0%, N = 299) and Airline 2 (20.9%, N = 250)—which are some of the largest airlines and, therefore, would be expected to show higher flight attendant representation in FADAP. However, some airlines were underrepresented in FADAP given their size[2] or for other reasons that are not clear. For example, one of the largest airlines,

---

[1]After a prepublication version of the report was provided to the FAA, this section was edited to anonymize the airline names.

[2]For more information, see Table A1 from FADAP Database Report in the Resources section of the report website.

TABLE 5-2 Characteristics of 1,196 Unique Flight Attendants Who Took Part in FADAP

Characteristic	Unique Flight Attendants (N = 1,196)
Age at first contact, mean (standard deviation)	44.4 (11.6)
Biological sex, N (%)[a]	
Female	686 (57.5)
Male	507 (42.5)
Airline, N (%)	
Airline 1	299 (25.0)
Airline 2	250 (20.9)
Airline 3	96 (8.0)
Airline 4	96 (8.0)
Airline 5	90 (7.5)
Airline 6	69 (5.8)
Airline 7	58 (4.8)
Airline 8	46 (3.8)
Airline 9	37 (3.1)
Other	155 (13.0)

NOTE: [a]Three flight attendants were missing data for biological sex.
SOURCE: Data from FADAP database and results from committee's "Call for Perspectives."

Airline 10, with 92,459 full-time employees in October 2022, was the most underrepresented in FADAP. Only 10 Airline 10 flight attendants took part in FADAP, which represents 0.01 percent of all Airline 10's full-time employees and 0.84 percent of the 1,196 flight attendants in the FADAP database.[3]

FADAP Treatment Episode Details

Table 5-3 shows treatment episode details as reported by treatment providers in the "Primary Treatment Summary" survey. Notably, the unit of analysis is now treatment episodes (N = 1,172), and not flight attendants, because some flight attendants (11.6% [N = 139 of 1,196 unique flight attendants]) had more than one treatment episode recorded in the database. Only treatment episodes for which a treatment provider reported both

---

[3]Information was pulled directly from an airline's website, but the FAA requested to anonymous all airlines.

TABLE 5-3 Treatment-Provider-Reported Treatment Details for the 1,172 FADAP Treatment Episodes

Episode Characteristic	Treatment Episodes (N = 1,172)[a] N (%)
Broad Treatment Issue	
Alcohol and mental health	574 (51.7)
Alcohol, drugs, and mental health	203 (18.3)
Alcohol only	166 (15.0)
Drugs and mental health	79 (7.1)
Mental health only	41 (3.7)
Alcohol and drugs	31 (2.8)
Drugs only	16 (1.4)
Specific Treatment Issue[b]	
Alcohol	921 (78.6)
Depression	519 (44.3)
Anxiety	419 (35.8)
Stimulants	124 (10.6)
PTSD	112 (9.6)
Sedatives	109 (9.3)
Cannabis	62 (5.3)
Opioids	49 (4.2)
Cocaine	49 (4.2)
Bipolar disorder	42 (3.6)
ADHD	30 (2.6)
Other mental health	118 (10.1)
Other drug abuse	20 (1.7)
Specific Medication-Assisted Treatments Offered	
Yes	819 (92.6)
No	65 (7.4)
Treatment Completed	
Yes	994 (92.0)
No	87 (8.0)
Treatment Length (days), median (IQR[c])	31 (29, 43)

NOTES: [a]Due to missing data, Ns ranged from 884 to 1,172 treatment episodes. [b]Specific treatment issues are not mutually exclusive because treatment episodes could involve more than one specific issue. Therefore, percentages do not sum to 100. [c]IQR = interquartile range. SOURCE: Data from FADAP database and results from committee's "Call for Perspectives."

admission and discharge dates are reported (N = 1,172). Due to missing data on some questions, analytic Ns ranged from 884 to 1,172 treatment episodes.

Approximately half of treatment episodes involved treatment for alcohol and mental health problems (51.7%, N = 574 of 1,110 treatment episodes). Almost one-third of treatment episodes (29.6%, N = 329 of 1,110 treatment episodes) involved treatment for a drug-use problem. Mental health problems were a common focus of treatment, particularly depression and anxiety, which were recognized by treatment providers as concerns in 44.3 percent (N = 519) and 35.8 percent (N = 419) of treatment episodes, respectively.

Medication-assisted treatment was offered in 92.6 percent of treatment episodes (N = 819 of 884 treatment episodes).[4] Treatment was completed in 92.0 percent of treatment episodes (N = 994 of 1,081 treatment episodes). The median length of treatment was 31 days (interquartile range = 29, 43).

FADAP Effectiveness and Satisfaction

Table 5-4 shows flight attendants' self-reported "recovery" status and satisfaction with FADAP at one year after treatment completion. The unit of analysis is treatment episodes. Treatment episodes with a discharge date by October 31, 2021, were considered eligible for the one-year follow-up survey (N = 990), given that the database was received in November 2022. Due to high rates of nonresponse by flight attendants to the one-year survey, analytic Ns ranged from 211 to 243 (i.e., 21.3–24.5% of 990 eligible episodes). Given the small N and limited ability to compare nonresponders and responders, there is a high degree of uncertainty about selection or attrition bias.

Flight attendants reported currently being in "recovery" at one-year post-treatment for 97.6 percent (N = 206) of treatment episodes and not in recovery for 2.4 percent (N = 5) of treatment episodes. Notably, this finding is based on only 211 (21.3%) of 990 eligible treatment episodes due to high rates of nonresponse to the one-year survey. Of the treatment episodes for which flight attendants reported being in recovery (N = 206), 95.6 percent (N = 197) were in continuous recovery for at least 30 days. Of the 197 treatment episodes that were in continuous recovery for at least 30 days, 68.3 percent (N = 125) of the episodes were characterized by a report of returning to work at one-year post-treatment.

---

[4]Note that ~25 percent of the 1,172 treatment episodes (N = 288) were missing data on whether medication-assisted treatment was offered. FADAP revised the question about medication-assisted treatment in 2020, and when data from 2020 onward were used, medication-assisted treatment was offered in 83.9 percent of treatment episodes (256 of 305).

TABLE 5-4 Flight Attendant-Reported Recovery and Return-to-Work Status and Satisfaction with FADAP at One-Year Post-Treatment for 990 Treatment Episodes Eligible for the One-Year Post-Treatment Survey

Outcome	Treatment Episodes (N = 990)[a] N (%)
Recovery Status[b]	
In recovery	206 (97.6)
Not in recovery	5 (2.4)
Returned to Work (among N = 197 in continuous recovery for at least 30 days)[c]	
Yes	125 (68.3)
No	58 (31.7)
Program Satisfaction[d]	
Recommend FADAP	215 (88.5)
I would use FADAP again	211 (86.8)
I am satisfied with FADAP	197 (81.1)
FADAP peer assistance made it possible to ask for help	203 (83.5)
Without FADAP, I would not have made it into treatment	203 (83.5)

NOTES: [a]The analyses are limited to 990 treatment episodes that were eligible for the one-year follow-up survey based on discharge date by October 31, 2021. Due to high rates of nonresponse among flight attendants with eligible treatment episodes, analytic Ns ranged from 211 to 243, with the exception of the analysis of return to work. [b]Flight attendants were asked: "Would you describe yourself as currently being in recovery from both alcohol and drugs of abuse?" [c]The question about return to work was asked only of the flight attendants who reported being in continuous recovery for at least 30 days. [d]Shows responses of "agree" or "strongly agree" on a five-point Likert scale.
SOURCE: Data from FADAP database and results from committee's "Call for Perspectives."

In terms of satisfaction with FADAP at one-year after treatment discharge, satisfaction ratings were high and ranged from 81.1 to 88.5 percent reporting "agree" or "strongly agree" to statements such as "I would use FADAP again" on a five-point scale ranging from "strongly disagree" to "strongly agree." However, the analytic N for satisfaction with FADAP ratings was 243 of 990 eligible episodes (24.5% of eligible episodes).

Approximately 16 percent of all unique treatment episodes (N = 182) were relapse episodes, defined as treatment episodes that occurred at least 28 days after the discharge date of a previous treatment episode.

**Agreement of Findings: A Comparison Between
FADAP Annual Reports and the Independent Analysis**

Findings from the 2022 FADAP annual report, which reports on all data collected since 2014, were summarized and compared with findings from the independent analysis (Nordberg, 2023). There was general agreement on the findings. However, whereas the FADAP annual report concludes from the data that the program is effective, the committee's interpretation of the data is more cautious. Low response rates to the one-year follow-up survey could bias outcomes such as recovery, return to work, and satisfaction with FADAP in a healthier/more positive direction.

Findings from the "Call for Perspectives" and Qualitative Interviews

The National Academies of Sciences, Engineering, and Medicine Committee developed a tool for gathering lived experiences ("Call for Perspectives") and commissioned a qualitative study to understand the perspectives of flight attendants and pilots with regard to FADAP and HIMS, respectively. The National Academies of Sciences, Engineering, and Medicine contracted with Jennifer P. Wisdom (PhD, MPH, ABPP) of Wisdom Consulting to conduct the investigation. Here we summarize the results of the investigation. Wisdom's full report, including copies of the "Call for Perspectives" and interview guide, can be found in the "Resources" section on the report's website.

The "Call for Perspectives" is an online tool the committee used to gather lived experiences, posted on the National Academies' website and disseminated via social media and mailing lists. Additionally, the committee enlisted the help of FADAP, HIMS, the Air Line Pilots Association, International, and other contacts within aviation to directly invite flight attendants and pilots to complete the "Call for Perspectives." The committee recognizes this could have introduced selection bias into the results, but to ensure anonymity of the respondents, the link was not tracked. The "Call for Perspectives" asked about substance use and its relationship to airline industry culture, treatment initiation and recovery, and perspectives and recommendations on FADAP and HIMS. There were 1,188 respondents. Most "Call for Perspectives" respondents were flight attendants (99%, N = 1,173). Therefore, the results summarized here represent the views of flight attendants and not pilots.

The majority of respondents were women (69%, N = 812), and 27 percent were men (N = 322). (The remaining preferred not to answer [3%] or selected "non-binary/other.") Most respondents had been employed in the industry for more than 10 years (63%, N = 746). A substantial percentage of respondents had no familiarity with the FADAP (33%, N = 395).

Approximately seven percent (N = 80) of respondents reported having previously been, or were currently, enrolled in FADAP. More than half of respondents stated that they would use FADAP if they thought they had a substance use disorder (52%, N = 616), and most respondents said they would recommend the program to a friend (91%, N = 84).

Purposive sampling was used to select a subset of "Call for Perspectives" respondents who indicated their willingness to complete qualitative interviews (N = 265 respondents). The sampling strategy sought to ensure diversity in profession (i.e., flight attendant versus pilot), sex, employment duration, and experience with the FADAP. Initial interview requests were sent to 40 purposely selected individuals. Given low response rates and time limitations, ultimately all 265 individuals who agreed in the "Call for Perspectives" to be contacted were invited to interview. Thirty-six interviews were conducted, and 35 of 36 interviewees were flight attendants. Therefore, the results from qualitative interviews reflect the views of flight attendants and not pilots.

Most interviewees were women (67%, N = 24), and most had more than 10 years of experience in the industry (75%, N = 27). Approximately 72 percent (N = 26) of interviewees had personal experience with substance use problems (80% alcohol; 16% psychostimulants; 8% sedatives; 4% GHB [gamma hydroxybutyrate, a depressant drug used as an intoxicant]; and 4% marijuana [percentages do not sum to 100% because of use of multiple substances]), and the remainder (N = 10) were not personally in recovery and not reporting substance misuse but had knowledge of a colleague or relative with a substance use disorder. Of 26 interviewees who had experience with substance misuse, all were in recovery; one had taken part in FADAP, six obtained treatment before FADAP existed, six sought treatment through the company or union Employee Assistance Program program, and the others sought treatment through other means (N = 10) or were unsure of how they got into treatment (N = 2). Three of 10 not in recovery were serving in a union role; 15 of the 26 who indicated they were in recovery were serving on their airline's FADAP committee or in a union stewardship role. Several of the 11 individuals in recovery (out of the total of 26) who were not serving on these committees indicated a desire to serve. One interviewee entered treatment due to a positive U.S. Department of Transportation (DOT) test, whereas the others reported entering treatment voluntarily. Treatment was typically inpatient residential treatment followed by intensive outpatient treatment or mutual support groups. Several interviewees discussed hardships associated with returning to work and the need for greater treatment support on returning to work, especially to cope with triggers such as serving alcohol to passengers.

Interviewees identified aspects of working in the airline industry that increase risk for substance misuse, such as long hours, poor sleep, loneliness, a culture of heavy drinking, and access to alcohol on the airplane and at airports. Interviewees revealed that some flight attendants do not recognize that they have a drinking problem, and, although crewmates are often aware of the problem, crewmates are hesitant to report it. Random testing by the DOT and the rule about no alcohol consumption eight hours prior to flying were reported to be ineffective substance-use deterrents. Interviewees mentioned the need for education and self-assessments about risky drinking to facilitate early intervention and treatment seeking.

Respondents to the "Call for Perspectives" and to the qualitative interviews clearly articulated the need for FADAP. However, they mentioned barriers to using FADAP, including a lack of awareness of FADAP, concerns about confidentiality, substance use stigma, fear of loss of employment (some airlines have a "zero tolerance" policy), and the financial costs of treatment. Suggested ways to improve FADAP included increasing promotion of FADAP to increase awareness of the program, dispelling misinformation to promote voluntary enrollment, enacting more rigorous substance testing requirements, and strengthening aftercare programs.

FINDINGS FOR HIMS

Findings from the HIMS Database

No independent analysis of the HIMS database was undertaken, because the committee's repeated requests for access to the HIMS database were denied. HIMS' claims about program effectiveness are summarized below, but because the committee lacked access to the relevant data, the claims could not be validated. To the committee's knowledge, the claims have not been subjected to other third-party validation.

HIMS' Self-reported Findings

HIMS asserts that the program is effective. Two sources for these claims are the HIMS executive summary and the HIMS 2021 Advanced Topics Seminar. The executive summary, which is dated December 2013 and is available on the HIMS website,[5] states,

> From 1972 to 1975, 14 pilots were returned to work following diagnosis and treatment, but since 1975, through the HIMS process, well over 5,000 pilots have been treated and safely returned to the cockpit. Airline pilots have been safely returned to their former cockpit positions and maintained abstinence, 85 to 90 percent of the time.

---

[5]For more information, see https://himsprogram.com/wp-content/uploads/2021/04/ExecSummary.pdf

While the timeline of HIMS' recovery measurements is unknown, this reported recovery rate is relative to the U.S. general population overall lifetime recovery rate of 75 percent (Jones et al., 2020).

A more recent version of the executive summary is not available on the website (checked March 10, 2023), but the following key points are still claimed:[6]

1. Between 1975 and 2022, more than 12,000 pilots had been helped, treated, and returned to their cockpits.
2. Eight hundred pilots recovering from an alcohol problem had achieved an 85 percent long-term abstinence rate.
3. A cost-benefit analysis showed a $9 return for every $1 spent on treatment.
4. The program enhanced flight safety.

In addition to the HIMS executive summary, claims about HIMS effectiveness were made in the HIMS 2021 Advanced Topics Seminar. The 2021 Advanced Topics Seminar data are shown in Tables 5-5, 5-6, and 5-7 and are reproduced exactly.

The seminar presented results from the HIMS database comprising first-class cases (N = 1,510 pilots, N = 1,291 Special Issuance Authorization) for whom an Airman Medical Examiner completed a datasheet from April 2011 to August 2021. Notably, the 1,510 pilots represent only 12.6 percent of the total 12,000 pilots HIMS claims have been returned to the cockpit from 1975–2021.

Table 5-5 shows the age ranges of the pilots and relapse rates by age. Most pilots in the report were between 40 and 59 years of age (70%). The overall relapse rate was 14 percent, and relapse rates were highest among the age 40–59 group (~16%) and generally lowest among the youngest age group (ages 20–29, 6.4%). It is difficult to evaluate what the low relapse rate means as it is unclear how relapse was defined or ascertained.

Table 5-6 shows pilots' substance of choice and relapse rates by substance. Most pilots' substance of choice was alcohol (92.5%), and the relapse rate for pilots whose substance of choice was alcohol was 13.7 percent. By comparison, few pilots' substance of choice was opioids (2%), but the relapse rate for pilots whose substance of choice was opioids was 40 percent.

Table 5-7 shows how pilots entered HIMS. Most pilots entered HIMS through self-referral (28.4%) or through an off-duty driving under the influence (DUI) citation (24.1%), and a relatively small fraction of pilots (8.4%) entered HIMS through a positive drug test given by the DOT. It should be

---

[6]Ibid.

TABLE 5-5 HIMS Pilots' Ages and Relapse Rates by Age

Age	N (% of Total)	Relapse, N (% of Age Group)
20–29	47 (3.7)	NR (6.4)
30–39	264 (20.7)	NR (7.7)
40–49	393 (31.2)	NR (16.5)
50–59	488 (38.7)	NR (16.2)
60–64	70 (5.6)	NR (14.3)
65+	2 (0.2)	NR (0.0)
Total	1,261[a]	NR (14.0)

NOTE: HIMS = Human Intervention Motivational Study. NR = not reported. [a]Total N is shown in the HIMS presentation as 1,261, but actual N (based on summing pilots in each age category) is 1,264. Both Ns are under the number of pilots claimed to be in the database (N = 1,510 pilots, N = 1,291 Special Issuance Authorization).
SOURCE: Committee generated from the 2021 HIMS Advanced Topics Seminar (September 13–14, 2021, Denver, CO).

TABLE 5-6 HIMS Pilots' Substance of Choice and Relapse Rates by Substance of Choice

Substance of Choice	N (% of Total)	Relapse Rate, N (% of Choice Substance Group)
Alcohol	1,166 (92.5)	NR (13.7)
Cannabis	24 (1.9)	NR (8.3)
Cocaine	23 (1.8)	NR (17.4)
Opioid (non-spec)	25 (2.0)	NR (40.0)
Opioid (semi-syn)	2 (0.2)	NR (0.0)
Stimulants	6 (0.5)	NR (0.0)
Other	15 (1.20)	NR (0.7)

NOTE: HIMS = Human Intervention Motivational Study. NR = not reported. Non-spec = non-specific. Semi-syn = semi-synthetic.
SOURCE: Committee generated from the 2021 HIMS Advanced Topics Seminar (September 13–14, 2021, Denver, CO).

noted that although "self-referral" sometimes entails a pilot independently recognizing that they need treatment without being under any particular workplace pressure to enter treatment at that time, in other cases pilots are advised to refer themselves to HIMS after they reported an incident (e.g., a DUI) that placed their medical certificate at risk.

TABLE 5-7 HIMS Pilot Program Entry

Entry Mechanism	N (%)[a]
Self-referral	496 (28.4)
Driving Under the Influence Off Duty	421 (24.1)
Intervention	329 (18.9)
Other Intervention	184 (10.6)
DOT + Test[b]	147 (8.4)
TSA/Police	58 (3.3)
Company	26 (1.5)
HIMS Airman Medical Examiner	9 (0.5)
Family	22 (1.3)
Failed Monitored Abstinence	1 (NR)

NOTE: HIMS = Human Intervention Motivational Study. DOT = Department of Transportation. TSA = Transportation Security Administration. [a]These percentages are slightly off if the total N is assumed to be 1,692 pilots (the sum of pilots across entry mechanisms), which is greater than the sum total of pilots reported to be included in the database supported by the seminar. However, it is unclear whether pilots were allowed to be included in more than one entry mechanism category. [b]DOT Positive Drug Test.
SOURCE: Committee generated from the 2021 HIMS Advanced Topics Seminar (September 13–14, 2021, Denver, CO).

Findings from the "Call for Perspectives" and Qualitative Interviews

Almost no data were collected from pilots as part of the National Academies' "Call for Perspectives" tool to gather experiences (N = 15 pilots vs. 1,157 flight attendants) or as part of the National Academies' commissioned study involving qualitative interviews (N = 1 pilot vs. N = 35 flight attendants). Unlike FADAP, the committee never received indications that HIMS and its administering organization, Air Line Pilots Association, International, ever distributed the link or sought pilot participation. The data collected from a very few pilots are not reported separately here to preserve anonymity.

6

Summary Assessment: Conclusions and Recommendations

Prior to 1974, the Federal Aviation Administration (FAA) lacked a program to encourage pilots to seek treatment for substance use problems so they could return to work safely. With a grant from the National Institute on Alcohol Abuse and Alcoholism to the Air Line Pilots Association, International (ALPA), and in cooperation with the FAA and airlines, the Human Intervention Motivational Study (HIMS) was created to assess the viability of an occupational program for pilots with alcohol use problems. HIMS was intended to provide a comprehensive approach to treatment and recovery by emphasizing identification, intervention, diagnostic assessment, treatment, continuing care, and relapse assistance. The Flight Attendant Drug and Alcohol Program (FADAP) was established in 2010.

In response to a congressional mandate, this study committee was tasked with reviewing available information on HIMS and FADAP, including recommendations concerning possible changes to the programs and lessons provided for other drug and alcohol treatment programs in the transportation sector. As the committee began its work pursuing the areas of Congressional interest, there was a presumption advanced by the FAA and the Congressional sponsors of the study that HIMS and FADAP were model programs that could serve as the basis for other drug and alcohol treatment programs in the transportation sector. Early in the pursuit of the committee's charge three observations became clear: (1) that the lack of information made available to the committee, for reasons described in Chapter 1, would limit the ability of the committee to execute the charge; (2) what information was available to the committee created uncertainty regarding the claims about the success of the programs in addressing substance misuse among pilots and flight attendants; (3) that there was a dearth of current published research on substance misuse directly related to safety-sensitive professionals.

Therefore, the committee conducted a careful review of the science associated with modern evidence-based treatments for substance use problems and considered the unique circumstances that affect case identification and treatment approaches for people employed in general safety-sensitive professions. Although relying on indirect evidence about individuals in safety-sensitive professions, the committee could nevertheless, in its judgement, reasonably inform the management and implementation of programs for pilots and flight attendants. The committee conducted detailed analyses of data obtained on the FADAP. It also examined the publicly reported data from HIMS and assessed those data in light of what is known about the prevalence of substance use disorders among pilots and the processes for identifying pilots with such problems. This concluding chapter reviews the committee's study approach and challenges encountered, followed by a summary of key findings across thematic areas that led to each of the committee's conclusions and recommendations.

STUDY APPROACH AND PROCESS

After gathering information about the HIMS and FADAP histories and methods, the committee reviewed presentations and reports prepared by HIMS and FADAP and program administrators in an effort to assess program outcomes and determine the approaches to case identification and treatment in the context of the prevailing scientific evidence. To supplement and independently assess the findings from these sources of information, the committee requested access to HIMS and FADAP outcome databases for analyses by a statistical consultant hired for the study. Furthermore, the committee developed a tool for obtaining testimonials of the lived experiences of pilots and flight attendants experiencing substance misuse problems through a "Call for Perspectives" issued to pilots and flight attendants. Committee members and staff also attended annual meetings of the two programs, met with program administrators and stakeholders, and arranged for interviews of a small group of participants to gain additional first-hand qualitative information about the programs.

In reviewing the literature on the treatment of substance use disorders and consulting experts in the field, the committee documented the changes that have been taking place on the basis of the disease model of addiction. The methods employed by HIMS and FADAP could thus be compared with the state of the best practices for screening, assessing, and treating substance use disorders, while taking into account the special context of professionals in safety-sensitive occupations such as pilots and flight attendants.

During this process, the committee faced several challenges, particularly with respect to access to available data and other information, limiting its pursuit of the charge. The committee was nevertheless able to obtain enough information to reach a few conclusions about the two programs, leading to some limited recommendations on program improvements.

The remainder of this chapter presents a summary of the committee's findings, followed by its conclusions and recommendations. The committee prioritized findings it viewed as most helpful to aligning the treatment services and overall administration and management of programs for pilots and flight attendants with current evidence on effective treatment for substance use disorders and considerations for safety-sensitive professionals. While the committee identified a few areas in which current practices are at odds with received evidence, it also identified areas where the programs align well with current thinking regarding best practices, such as HIMS' and FADAP's emphasis on peer networks to support recovery.

The committee's conclusions and recommendations are aimed at processes that can improve the HIMS and FADAP. Because HIMS and FADAP differ in important ways that have implications for how they are, and perhaps should be, designed and assessed, the issues related to each are discussed separately as warranted. Because the committee's recommendations are intended to improve both program management and oversight, they are directed as appropriate to FAA (primarily through its Office of Aerospace Medicine, which is responsible for a broad range of medical programs and services for both the domestic and international aviation communities) and to Congress.

ALIGNING SUBSTANCE USE DISORDER PRACTICES AND POLICIES FOR HIMS AND FADAP WITH THE EVIDENCE BASE

The key functions that the committee sought to understand, and subsequently provide guidance on, related to the following questions: (a) How are pilots and flight attendants that misuse substances identified? (b) How do pilots and flight attendants that misuse substances and need treatment get engaged with treatment? (c) What is the content of treatment strategies employed by the two programs? And (d) How are flight attendants and pilots in need of follow-up care directed to appropriate and effective providers of care?

Before presenting the committee's individual summary findings, conclusions, and recommendations, the following observations should be highlighted. First, ensuring public safety while providing support for employees needing treatment is an important consideration that applies to all professions that have a duty to serve and protect the public. Throughout this consensus study, the committee was cognizant of the precarious balance in commercial aviation between ensuring public safety and meeting an obligation to help employees in safety-sensitive positions receive the treatment they need to address substance misuse and use disorders. The primary role and responsibility of FAA is public safety, and thus in many cases it could be reasonable to mandate different approaches to case identification and use of treatment settings than those common in care of the general population. The summary findings highlight some areas where employees could obtain better treatment for substance use disorders by aligning with current, evidence-based science while also minimizing risk to the public.[1]

Second, the implementation of substance misuse programs for pilots and flight attendants is highly decentralized, which has implications for the FAA's ability to track substance misuse and its treatment in pilots and flight attendants, and for the committee's conclusions and recommendations As described in Chapter 2, FAA follows regulations from the U.S. Department of Transportation (DOT) issued to implement statutory provisions that authorize DOT agencies to provide substance use disorder programs in the different transportation modes. It is the policies and procedures of FAA, then, that create the operational frameworks for HIMS' and FADAP's local execution by the airlines and relevant unions.

Third, the implementation of effective programs depends on the ability to assess and monitor practices and outcomes for appropriate management and oversight.

The remainder of this section reviews the specific findings, conclusions, and recommendations developed by the committee, which are informed by key features of evidence-based practices drawn from Chapter 3 and summarized in Box 6-1. The committee observed departures from these practices in its review of HIMS and FADAP in certain key thematic areas. These areas include:

- diagnosis and case identification;
- barriers to early help seeking and access to treatment;
- allowances and encouragement for individualized treatment; and
- use of evidence-based criteria in the selection of treatment programs.

The conclusions and recommendations are offered within each of these areas with the goal of identifying potential changes to HIMS and FADAP that could better align the programs with the current evidence base for substance use disorder programs and treatment. We reiterate that because published research on substance misuse among pilots or flight attendants,

---

[1] While this report focuses on substance misuse prevention, intervention, and treatment to algin with the statement of task, the committee fully acknowledges that the FAA's primary responsibility is ensuring the safety of the national airspace.

BOX 6-1
Committee-Identified Key Features of Evidence-Based Practices

Diagnosis and Case Identification
- Workplace policies that promote early identification and treatment
- Evidence-based screening tools and assessment models
- Diagnostic procedures and policies that use the most recent evidence-based definitions of substance use disorders (currently *Diagnostic and Statistical Manual of Mental Disorders, Fifth Edition*) and align with the most current clinical evidence

Removing Barriers to Identification and Treatment
- Increasing awareness of substance use disorder programs
- Decreasing stigma around mental illness and substance use disorders
- Reducing as much as appropriate the fear of retaliation and of threat of termination

Individualized Treatment Allowances
- Identification of levels of care and treatment options that are based on an individual's unique clinical presentation
- Lengths of stay that are based on an individual's needs and strengths

Selecting Treatment Programs
- Programs that use approaches supported by scientifically valid empirical data
- Programs that offer cohort care and providers who are highly skilled, credentialed in evidence-based treatments, and experienced in treating professionals in safety-sensitive occupations

---

or even safety-sensitive professionals, is lacking, these conclusions and recommendations are based primarily on evidence from the robust literature available on the qualities of effective substance use programs in general that, in the committee's judgement, are sufficiently generalizable across individuals and contexts to be able to reasonably inform the management and implementation of programs for pilots and flight attendants, while noting special considerations that could apply to the aviation context.

Diagnosis and Case Identification

The committee observed that current definitions for substance use disorders in the Code of Federal Regulations (CFR) do not always align with current science-based approaches to diagnosis. For example, the FAA's language and diagnostic criteria for differentiating between substance abuse and substance dependence (as defined by 14 CFR § 67.107 and reviewed in Chapter 2 of this report) are more restrictive than those in the *Diagnostic and Statistical Manual of Mental Disorders, Fifth Edition* [DSM-5]. The FAA also uses different blood alcohol content thresholds. This can lead to a pilot meeting the FAA definition of substance abuse or dependence but not the clinical DSM-5 criteria for a substance use disorder.

It is understandable that for the sake of public safety, the primary duty written into its legal charter, the FAA may choose to apply additional considerations in defining what is acceptable substance use for the purpose of case identification. However, while full alignment with DSM criteria may not always be feasible without increasing significant operational risks, more consistent application of evidence-based diagnostic practices could better align treatment approaches with the current science.

Conclusion: The Federal Aviation Administration needs to apply the criteria of the Diagnostic and Statistical Manual of Mental Disorders more consistently to its policies for better alignment with an evidence-based approach to diagnosis and decisions about course of treatment as appropriate to the aviation context.

Recommendation 1: The Federal Aviation Administration should revise sections of the Code of Federal Regulations (CFR), especially 14 CFR Part 67 (Medical Standards and Certification), to align, to the extent reasonable in the aviation setting, with the most current evidence-based diagnostic approaches for substance use disorders that consider illness severity and lead to more personalized treatment.

Barriers to Early Help Seeking and Access to Affordable Treatment

Even when substance misuse treatment is available, there are often several barriers that keep aviation workers from accessing the services they need. These can come in the form of keeping individuals from even seeking help, due to concerns about employer retaliation, loss of employment, or general stigma related to substance use and mental illness. They may also be more structural barriers, such as lack of financial access or ability to pay for the treatment offered.

Some barriers are inherent to the context of the aviation industry, however, and public safety concerns may preclude their removal. But other barriers can be addressed by cultivating a climate that is supportive of employees' overall well-being and participation in available programs where appropriate. For example, strict, nonconfidential reporting requirements for mental health and substance use disorders, and the subsequent threat of employment consequences stemming from beginning treatment, can discourage and deter early treatment. Such requirements can especially affect flight attendants given their weaker employment attachments relative to those of pilots. Additionally, HIMS requires an open release of information (ROI) to be shared with them, allowing access to all records from a treatment episode. While this ensures that employees remain in compliance, it also discourages the initial disclosure of said information, as employees are concerned about losing their careers. Limiting ROIs or placing parameters on which information is shared could increase confidentiality of the employee during their treatment while ensuring a safe return to work. An ideal practice would be to encourage help-seeking by offering access to confidential, voluntary mental health and substance use treatment.

A significant barrier for pilots entering substance use disorder treatment is the unique medical certification requirements that pilots must meet. While HIMS does offer the prospect of a return to the flightdeck upon completion of treatment, identification of a co-occurring disqualifying condition places the pilot's medical certificate and, in turn, the pilot's career and livelihood at risk. The committee found a lack of opportunity for prevention or early intervention through confidential sharing of information about health and well-being. Aside from policies that have direct impacts on employment, developing policies that cultivate a climate of help-seeking and health-promoting environments can also contribute to reducing barriers to treatment. For example, creating a context that avoids stigmatizing people with substance use disorders supports voluntary reporting and early treatment, including use of specific nonstigmatizing language. Because screening for substance misuse and comorbid conditions during annual physical exams is known to help to identify misuse, and because existing screenings are yielding rates of 0.5 percent from aviation medical examiners (AME's) annual examinations, when general screening rates are typically greater than 14 percent, attention is needed to make the AME screening more rigorous and reliable.

Additionally, a key component of an effective program is ensuring awareness of the program. Responses that the committee received from both flight attendants and pilots indicated that many are perhaps unaware of FADAP or HIMS until they have a serious substance use disorder. Without knowledge that the program exists, it will be difficult to get employees the help they need or have them be willing to come forward and be transparent about their concerns or situation.

Conclusion: Opportunities could be better leveraged to mitigate barriers to early identification, help seeking, and treatment, and to provide access to affordable treatment.

Recommendation 2: The Federal Aviation Administration should ensure that mandated annual physical exams (e.g., aviation medical examiner examination) for all safety-sensitive professions require screening for substance misuse use tools that are validated for the population and setting.

Recommendation 3: While employment termination is a legitimate outcome if return-to-work policies are not met, the Federal Aviation Administration should ensure that airlines identify and remove features of their workplace substance misuse policies and procedures that are likely barriers to early identification and treatment, such as disclosures that are not likely related to performance in a safety-sensitive position, and consider opportunities to promote more fully early identification and treatment.[2]

- This committee recognizes the FAA's expectation of complete transparency from pilots about their physical and mental health to ensure the safety of the public and the national airspace. We also recognize, however, that this requirement may lead pilots to avoid accessing care that is observable to the airlines and to the FAA, and/or lead to dishonest reporting on their Form 8500-8 to avoid jeopardizing their medical certification, and thereby their ability to fly. Such behavior, however, likely serves to increase the risk of adverse events. Thus, while we acknowledge that full implementation of the recommendation may not be immediately actionable until policies and procedures are in place to mitigate concerns about potential short-term risks to operational impairment, the recommended actions remain worthy of serious consideration by the FAA in meeting the ultimate goals of public safety and pilot health.
- As examples for implementation:
    - The FAA could consider not requiring the release of a pilot's full record as part of medical certification. If concerns for disqualifying conditions are present for a particular pilot (e.g., suicidal ideation, psychosis, ADHD, bipolar disorder), a full release of records could still be required.
    - Because mental health issues co-occur with substance use disorders, the FAA could encourage pilots to confidentially (barring a diagnosis of a major disqualifying condition) seek early care for mental health issues, potentially through a limited waiver for Form 8500-8 or their airline's EAP.

---

[2]After a prepublication version of the report was provided to the FAA, this section was clarified to accurately reflect FAA's authorities.

— The FAA could update Form 8500-8 to be more encouraging of treatment-seeking by not requiring the dates and reasons for mental health visits and asking whether the pilot has sought mental health care (yes/no).

Financial Barriers

In addition to policies and culture, the decentralized structure of HIMS and FADAP results in great variability in the financial costs faced by aviation workers, with flight attendants usually facing greater liabilities that serve to create barriers to care. Although goals and FAA special issuance authorization standards are consistent, the program implementation varies among airlines. Pilots employed by major carriers with robust collective bargaining agreements and union support will often be provided with stronger financial support. Smaller carriers with more limited budgets may leave pilots with much more limited financial protection for mandated treatment and required evaluations and limited financial support during the medical leave.

Flight attendants are more likely than pilots to have limited funding sources to pay for treatment. Moreover, the decision of a flight attendant to go into treatment extends beyond the actual expenses incurred in treatment. Most flight attendants are treated in residential care programs, which in addition to being a high-cost modality results in extended absence from work and income loss.

Conclusion: Airlines and unions are central to the implementation of the testing programs and management of the Human Intervention and Motivational Study and Flight Attendant Drug and Alcohol Program programs. The discretion that airlines and unions possess results in much heterogeneity in program operations and employees' access to financial support for treatment.

Conclusion: Improved financial protection against treatment costs and income losses, for flight attendants in particular, would help ensure they can receive the full range of appropriate treatment to address their clinical needs. Without this change and parity in access to affordable evidence-based coverage across airlines, flight attendants may suffer significant economic losses.

Recommendation 4: Commercial airline carriers should ensure affordable access for mental health and substance misuse-related services for pilots and flight attendants consistent with the Mental Health Parity and Addiction Equity Act.

Allowances and Encouragement for Individualized Treatment

Currently, regardless of diagnosis, HIMS and FADAP emphasize 30 days of residential treatment over individualized treatment plans based on multidimensional assessment. While that is consistent with American Society of Addiction Medicine (ASAM) best practice recommendations for professionals in safety-sensitive occupations and treatment practices for physicians involved with physician health programs, other effective, more flexible, and less costly treatment modalities may be more appropriate. For some, 30 days of residential treatment may not be adequate. Level-of-care placement decisions are insufficiently linked to the severity of illness and individual circumstances. The benefits and risks of any medical treatment must be weighed before the treatment proceeds; this principle applies, of course, to the use of medications for addiction treatment in the context of professionals working in safety-sensitive occupations. However, it is unclear what process the FAA and other oversight organizations for pilots, flight attendants, and other professionals in safety-sensitive occupations use to evaluate and mitigate the risk associated with medication for addiction treatment.

Furthermore, although many mutual help groups exist, Alcoholics Anonymous (AA) is typically the most researched and has the most evidence on its impact on outcomes. HIMS and FADAP continue to recommend AA engagement specifically for their participants. However, that decision may alienate some employees given AA's spiritual nature and undertones.[3] Some evidence shows that other mutual help groups can be just as effective as AA, and other research has shown that social connections with like-minded peers and the adaptive, community-based system they provide are often responsible for treatment benefits.

Conclusion: By supporting an individualized approach to treatment, the Federal Aviation Administration could better align treatment options for pilots and flight attendants with an evidence-based approach.

Recommendation 5: Administrators of both the Human Intervention and Motivational Study and the Flight Attendant Drug and Alcohol Program, with the support of the Federal Aviation Administration, should encourage and support individualized treatment and continuing care programs based on the severity of the individual pilot or flight attendant's substance misuse and that person's preferences.

---

[3]Captain Dave Fielding, British Airways, presentation to the committee, November 1, 2022, that included an overview of substance use disorder and mental health support systems in UK aviation as a comparison to HIMS.

The following elements should be considered in implementing the recommendation:

- A determination of the severity of disease and treatment recommendations should be made by addiction experts using the ASAM dimensions and should include collateral information. Assessment should include consideration of what puts someone at higher risk (e.g., onset of use, family history of substance use, trauma history) and objective measures of substance use and screening for co-occurring physical and mental health conditions.
- Treatment recommendations, including level of care and length of stay, should be based on the severity of the disease and individual circumstances, not dictated by a required 30 days of residential treatment.
- Aeromedically significant deficits are of significant concern for pilots and the safety of the airspace. Current science indicates that there are medication-assisted treatment (MAT) options that could provide significant benefit to preventing relapse while posing minimal risk for impairment, particularly with appropriate medication selection and monitoring, and as a result of the required neurocognitive evaluations for pilots involved with HIMS. The FAA has a model for successfully and safely introducing lifesaving mental health medications that improve the safety of the airspace; they should explore how this could be adapted for MAT.
- Aftercare planning should, at minimum, include peer support and offer nonspiritual options beyond AA, while being transparent on the depth of the evidence base for these different voluntary involvement programs.

Use of Evidence-Based Criteria in the Selection of Treatment Programs

Each airline has substantial autonomy and discretion in the treatment options it chooses to offer under the auspices of HIMS and FADAP. Although several airlines engage the same treatment programs or models of treatment, local discretion results in providing a range of inconsistent treatment options. While such variation is not necessarily a problem, the justification for the selection of treatment programs is not clearly set forth. One consideration is the differences in the ability of different airlines—from major carriers to smaller, regional carriers—to provide financial incentives and support for effective treatments. As discussed previously, the committee acknowledges that the different levels of financial support offered by the airline would need to be addressed to ensure more widespread involvement and participation in HIMS and FADAP.

Conclusion: The implementation of Title 14, Part 67 of the Code of Federal Regulations needs to be more consistent among airline carriers regarding employee benefits, support structures, and access to effective treatment options.

Recommendation 6: National Human Intervention and Motivational Study (HIMS) and Flight Attendant Drug and Alcohol Program (FADAP) organizations should provide clear criteria that follow from evidence on effective treatment for the selection and approval of treatment settings to which each airline's HIMS/FADAP can make referrals.

In implementing this last recommendation, the key features of evidence-based practice previously mentioned in Box 6-1 should be considered when establishing criteria for the selection of effective substance use disorder treatment programs for transportation professionals.

QUALITY OF DATA AND DATA ANALYSIS FOR PROGRAM MANAGEMENT AND DECISION-MAKING

In its review, the committee encountered several areas where information is lacking that is necessary for the adequate assessment of program functions and performance. Effective programs depend on the ability of the FAA and Congress to assess and monitor practices and performance in the services of appropriate management and oversight. As detailed in Chapter 1, the committee experienced challenges with accessing data and uncovered evidence that raised concerns about the quality of data available to the FAA about the programs, suggesting potential limitations on the quality and comprehensiveness of data available to Congress and the FAA for them to fulfill their management and oversight roles.

HIMS and the FAA make claims about the success of the program that could not be substantiated by the committee, and the committee's review of reports available to the public raised concerns about important elements of the program that could not be addressed with available information. In several instances data pointed to failure of processes that are inconsistent with claims of success. The lack of meaningful referral based on the annual medical examination of pilots noted earlier is a case in point. ALPA, the administrator of HIMS, acknowledges that the database is limited in its ability to produce advanced insights,[4] which seems inconsistent with many public statements on the HIMS website that include findings from data on HIMS. As an example of an important issue that could not be fully examined, the committee was unable to discern to what degree there is unmet

---

[4]For more information, see Appendix D.

need and the potential reasons for it. It appears, from the data available, that a sizable portion of pilots likely to have a substance use disorder do not access treatment through HIMS. Alternatively, pilots who need and are seeking treatment may be accessing it outside of the federally mandated system of treatment and return-to-work requirements. HIMS treats roughly 1.5 percent of pilots, yet by HIMS' own unconfirmed estimates the prevalence rate among pilots for having a substance use disorder is between 8 and 12 percent, which would be lower than the 13 to 15 percent derived from the research literature.[5] The troubling implication of this is that the FAA and Congress have limited visibility of the degree to which pilots with substance misuse problems are being treated.

Likewise, the FADAP has major gaps in addressing substance misuse and substance use disorders for many flight attendants employed by U.S. commercial airlines. The analysis of the FADAP database highlighted data quality issues that limited the committee's ability to assess program operations. Specifically, many flight attendants were lost to follow-up tracking and fewer than half of expected flight attendants were captured in the data, because data from some major airlines were missing. This resulted in clear geographic distortions and likely demographic distortions relative to the overall population of flight attendants.

Conclusion: The committee observed issues with data quality and data access, both of which hinder the ability to assess, manage, and oversee substance use programs.

Recommendation 7: In the service of effective oversight and continuous improvement of the Human Intervention Motivational Study (HIMS) and based on our analysis of the Flight Attendant Drug and Alcohol Program (FADAP) database, the Federal Aviation Administration (FAA) should require that FADAP collect and maintain more reliable and complete data. Based on the lack of independent analysis of the HIMS database, the FAA should require that HIMS collect and maintain reliable and complete data. Data collected for both programs should at minimum include the number of pilots and flight attendants who contact them, the number of pilots and flight attendants referred for treatment, patterns and components of treatment, and long-term post-treatment outcomes.

In implementing the recommendation:
- The parties responsible for collecting and managing data on HIMS and FADAP should be required to adhere to specified standards

---

[5]https://himsprogram.com/

for data collection and to include specific post-treatment outcome measures and follow-up assessments to ensure that more complete data are collected.

- In the service of reviewing overall program effectiveness, deidentified data records that HIMS and FADAP collect should be able to be linked to the DOT's testing database and easily exported to allow more useful and transparent reporting to Congress and any other delegated independent auditors, a process that includes anonymization of data.[6]
- HIMS and FADAP should be required to report to the FAA how they are analyzing and using the data they collect to inform internal program improvements and external customer satisfaction in compliance with EO 13642 and EO 14058. For example, HIMS should consider adopting FADAP's practice of compiling and publishing an annual, detailed database report.

---

[6]After a prepublication version of the report was provided to the FAA, this section was edited to clarify the specific database and note the type of data records.

References

Acevedo, A., Panas, L., Garnick, D., Acevedo-Garcia, D., Miles, J., Ritter, G., & Campbell, K. (2018). Disparities in the treatment of substance use disorders: Does where you live matter? *Journal of Behavioral Health Services & Research*, 45(4), 533–549. https://doi.org/10.1007/s11414-018-9586-y

Alcoholics Anonymous. (2002). *Alcoholics Anonymous: Big book* (4th ed.).

Althubaiti A. (2016). Information bias in health research: Definition, pitfalls, and adjustment methods. *Journal of Multidisciplinary Healthcare*, 9, 211–217. https://doi.org/10.2147/JMDH.S104807

American Psychiatric Association (APA). (2020). *Task force on psychological assessment and evaluation guidelines.* https://www.apa.org/about/policy/guidelines-psychological-assessment-evaluation.pdf

———. (2022). *Diagnostic and statistical manual of mental disorders* (5th ed.). https://doi.org/10.1176/appi.books.9780890425787

American Society of Addiction Medicine. (n.d.). *The ASAM criteria: Evidence base.* https://www.asam.org/asam-criteria/about-the-asam-criteria/evidence-base

Anda, R. F., Felitti, V. J., Bremner, J. D., Walker, J. D., Whitfield, C., Perry, B. D., Dube, S. R., & Giles, W. H. (2006). The enduring effects of abuse and related adverse experiences in childhood: A convergence of evidence from neurobiology and epidemiology. *European Archives of Psychiatry and Clinical Neuroscience*, 256(3), 174–186. https://doi.org/10.1007%2Fs00406-005-0624-4

Andresen, M., Domsch, M. E., & Cascorbi, A. H. (2007). Working unusual hours and its relationship to job satisfaction: A study of European maritime pilots. *Journal of Labor Research*, 28, 714–734. https://doi.org/10.1007/s12122-007-9010-5

Arboleda, A., Morrow, P. C., Crum, M. R., & Shelley, M. C., 2nd (2003). Management practices as antecedents of safety culture within the trucking industry: Similarities and differences by hierarchical level. *Journal of Safety Research*, 34(2), 189–197. https://doi.org/10.1016/s0022-4375(02)00071-3

Atherton, M. J. (2019). Alcohol and other substance abuse assessment. In R. Bor, C. Eriksen, T. P. Hubbard, & R. King (Eds.), *Pilot Selection* (pp. 205–212). CRC Press https://doi.org/10.4324/9780429492105

Bahji, A., D. Crockford, & El-Guebaly, N. (2022). Neurobiology and symptomatology of post-acute alcohol withdrawal: A mixed-studies systematic review. *Journal of Studies on Alcohol and Drugs, 83*(4), 461–469.

Baldisseri M. R. (2007). Impaired healthcare professional. *Critical Care Medicine, 35*(2 Suppl), S106–S116. https://doi.org/10.1097/01.CCM.0000252918.87746.96

Bandura, A. (1982). Self-efficacy mechanism in human agency. *American Psychologist, 37*(2), 122–47. https://doi.org/10.1037/0003-066X.37.2.122

Barata, I. A., Shandro, J. R., Montgomery, M., Polansky, R., Sachs, C. J., Duber, H. C., Weaver, L. M., Heins, A., Owen, H. S., Josephson, E. B., & Macias-Konstantopoulos, W. (2017). Effectiveness of SBIRT for alcohol use disorders in the emergency department: A systematic review. *The Western Journal of Emergency Medicine, 18*(6), 1143–1152. https://doi.org/10.5811/westjem.2017.7.34373

Bates, M. E., Buckman, J. F., & Nguyen, T. T. (2013). A role for cognitive rehabilitation in increasing the effectiveness of treatment for alcohol use disorders. *Neuropsychology Review, 23*(1), 27–47. https://doi.org/10.1007/s11065-013-9228-3

Beaulieu, M., Tremblay, J., Baudry, C., Pearson, J., & Bertrand, K. (2021). A systematic review and meta-analysis of the efficacy of the long-term treatment and support of substance use disorders. *Social Science & Medicine, 285*, 114289.

Becker, H. C. (1998). Kindling in alcohol withdrawal. *Alcohol Health and Research World, 22*(1), 25–33. https://pubs.niaaa.nih.gov/publications/arh22-1/25-34.pdf

Bone, C., Gelberg, L., Vahidi, M., Leake, B., Yacenda-Murphy, J., & Andersen, R. M. (2016). Under-reporting of risky drug use among primary care patients in federally qualified health centers. *Journal of Addiction Medicine, 10*(6), 387–394. https://doi.org/10.1097/ADM.0000000000000246

Botch, S. R., & Johnson, R. D. (2009). Antiemetic and sedative levels found together in 26 civil aviation pilot fatalities, 2000-2006. *Aviation, Space, and Environmental Medicine, 79*(6). https://doi.org/10.3357/asem.2274.2008

Bouza, C., Angeles, M., Muñoz, A., & Amate, J. M. (2004). Efficacy and safety of naltrexone and acamprosate in the treatment of alcohol dependence: A systematic review. *Addiction, 99*(7), 811–828.

Boyd, J. W., & Knight, J. R. (2012). Ethical and managerial considerations regarding state physician health programs. *Journal of Addiction Medicine, 6*(4), 243–246. https://doi.org/10.1097/ADM.0b013e318262ab09

Brown, A.D. (2015). Identities and identity work. *International Journal of Management Reviews, 17*, 20–40. https://doi.org/10.1111/ijmr.12035

Bureau of Labor Statistics (BLS). (2022a). *Occupational employment and wages, May 2022: 53-2012 commercial pilots.* https://www.bls.gov/oes/current/oes532012.htm

———. (2022b). *Occupational outlook handbook, airline and commercial pilots.* https://www.bls.gov/ooh/transportation-and-material-moving/airline-and-commercial-pilots.htm

———. (2023). *Occupational employment and wages, May 2022: 53-2031 flight attendants.* https://www.bls.gov/oes/current/oes532031.htm

Butcher, J. N. (2002). Assessing pilots with 'the wrong stuff: A call for research on emotional health factors in commercial aviators. *International Journal of Selection and Assessment, 10*(1–2), 168–184. https://doi.org/10.1111/1468-2389.00204

Cantor, J. H., DeYoreo, M., Hanson, R., Kofner, A., Kravitz, D., Salas, A., Stein, B. D., & Kapinos, K. A. (2022). Patterns in geographic distribution of substance use disorder treatment facilities in the US and accepted forms of payment from 2010 to 2021. *JAMA Network Open, 5*(11), e2241128.

Castells, X., Kosten, T. R., Capellà, D., Vidal, X., Colom, J., & Casas, M. (2009). Efficacy of opiate maintenance therapy and adjunctive interventions for opioid dependence with comorbid cocaine use disorders: A systematic review and meta-analysis of controlled clinical trials. *The American Journal of Drug and Alcohol Abuse, 35*(5), 339–349.

Cheetham, A., Picco, L., Barnett, A., Lubman, D. I., & Nielsen, S. (2022). The impact of stigma on people with opioid use disorder, opioid treatment, and policy. *Substance Abuse and Rehabilitation, 13*, 1–12. https://doi.org/10.2147/sar.S304566

Clark, R. E. (2001). Family support and substance use outcomes for persons with mental illness and substance use disorders. *Schizophrenia Bulletin, 27*(1), 93–101. https://doi.org/10.1093/oxfordjournals.schbul.a006862

Cleland, J. G. F., Torp-Pedersen, C., Coletta, A. P., & Lammiman, M. J. (2004), A method to reduce loss to follow-up in clinical trials: Informed, withdrawal of consent. *European Journal of Heart Failure, 6*, 1–2.

Connock, M., Juarez-Garcia, A., Jowett, S., Frew, E., Liu, Z., Taylor, R. J., Fry-Smith, A., Day, E., Lintzeris, N., Roberts, T., Burls, A., & Taylor, R. S. (2007). Methadone and buprenorphine for the management of opioid dependence: A systematic review and economic evaluation. *Health Technology Assessment, 11*(9).

Corrigan, P., Schomerus, G., Shuman, V., Kraus, D., Perlick, D., Harnish, A., Kulesza, M., Kane-Willis, K., Qin, S., & Smelson, D. (2017). Developing a research agenda for understanding the stigma of addictions: Part I: Lessons from the mental health stigma literature. *The American Journal on Addictions, 26*(1), 59–66. https://doi.org/10.1111/ajad.12458

Coviello, D. M., Zanis, D. A., Wesnoski, S. A., Palman, N., Gur, A., Lynch, K. G., & McKay, J. R. (2013). Does mandating offenders to treatment improve completion rates? *Journal of Substance Abuse Treat, 44*(4), 417–425. https://doi.org/10.1016/j.jsat.2012.10.003

Cullen, P., Cahill, J., & Gaynor, K. (2021). A qualitative study exploring well-being and the potential impact of work-related stress among commercial airline pilots. *Aviation Psychology and Applied Human Factors, 11*, 11–12. https://doi.org/10.1027/2192-0923/a000199

DeFulio, A., Donlin, W. D., Wong, C. J., & Silverman, K. (2009). Employment-based abstinence reinforcement as a maintenance intervention for the treatment of cocaine dependence: A randomized controlled trial. *Addiction, 104*(9), 1530–1538. https://doi.org/10.1111/j.1360-0443.2009.02657.x

DeHoff, M. C., & Cusick, S. K. (2018). Mental health in commercial aviation-depression & anxiety of pilots. *International Journal of Aviation, Aeronautics, and Aerospace, 5*(5), 5. https://commons.erau.edu/ijaaa/vol5/iss5/5

Delaney-Black, V., Chiodo, L.M., Hannigan, J.H., Greenwald, M.K., Janisse, J., Patterson, G., Huestis, M.A., Ager, J., & Sokol, R.J. (2010). Just say "I don't": Lack of concordance between teen report and biological measures of drug use. *Pediatrics. 126*(5), 887–893. https://doi.org/10.1542/peds.2009-3059.

Department of Transportation. (2021). *2021 MIS data.* https://www.transportation.gov/odapc/2021-MIS-DATA

DuPont, R. L., Compton, W. M., & McLellan, A. T. (2015). Five-year recovery: A new standard for assessing effectiveness of substance usement disorder treatment. *Journal of Substance Abuse Treatment, 58*, 1–5

DuPont, R. L., McLellan, A. T., Carr, G., Gendel, M., & Skipper, G. E. (2009). How are addicted physicians treated? A national survey of physician health programs. *Journal of Substance Abuse Treatment, 37*(1), 1–7.

DuPont, R. L., & Merlo, L. (2018). Physician health programs: A model for treating substance use disorders. *The Judges Journal, 57*(1). https://ncphp.org/wp-content/uploads/2018/03/PHPs-A-Model.pdf

DuPont, R. L., & Skipper, G. E. (2012). Six lessons from state physician health programs to promote long-term recovery. *Journal of Psychoactive Drugs, 44*(1), 72–78. https://doi.org/10.1080/02791072.2012.660106

Edmondson, A. (1999). Psychological safety and learning behavior in work teams. *Administrative Science Quarterly, 44*(2), 350–383. https://doi.org/10.2307/2666999

Engel, G. L. (1977). The need for a new medical model: A challenge for biomedicine. *Science, 196*(4286), 129–136. https://doi.org/10.1126/science.847460

Evert, D. L., & Oscar-Berman, M. (1995). Alcohol-related cognitive impairments: An overview of how alcoholism may affect the workings of the brain. *Alcohol Health and Research World, 19*(2), 89–96.

Eylem, O., de Wit, L., van Straten, A., Steubl, L., Melissourgaki, Z., Danışman, G. T., de Vries, R., Kerkhof, A. J. F. M., Bhui, K., & Cuijpers, P. (2020). Stigma for common mental disorders in racial minorities and majorities a systematic review and meta-analysis. *BMC Public Health, 20*(1), 879. https://doi.org/10.1186/s12889-020-08964-3

Federal Aviation Administration. (2012, October 11). *Fitness for duty* [Advisory Circular No. 117-3]. https://www.faa.gov/documentLibrary/media/Advisory_Circular/AC%20117-3.pdf

———. (2023a). *U.S. civil airmen statistics.* https://www.faa.gov/data_research/aviation_data_statistics/civil_airmen_statistics

———. (2023b). *Guide for aviation medical examiners.* https://www.faa.gov/ame_guide

Feuer, B. (1987). Innovations in employee assistance programs: A case study at the Association of Flight Attendants. In Riley A. (ed.), *Occupational stress and organizational effectiveness.*

Fleury, M. J., Djouini, A., Huỳnh, C., Tremblay, J., Ferland, F., Ménard, J. M., & Belleville, G. (2016). Remission from substance use disorders: A systematic review and meta-analysis. *Drug and Alcohol Dependence, 168*, 293–306.

Food and Drug Administration (FDA). (n.d.). *Information about medication-assisted treatment (MAT).* https://www.fda.gov/drugs/information-drug-class/information-about-medication-assisted-treatment-mat

———. (2023). *Risk evaluation and mitigation strategies.* https://www.fda.gov/drugs/drug-safety-and-availability/risk-evaluation-and-mitigation-strategies-rems

Foster, D., & Ren, X. (2015). Work–family conflict and the commodification of women's employment in three Chinese airlines. *The International Journal of Human Resource Management, 26*(12), 1568–1585.

French, M. T., Popovici, I., & Tapsell, L. (2008). The economic costs of substance abuse treatment: Updated estimates and cost bands for program assessment and reimbursement. *Journal of Substance Abuse Treatment, 35*(4), 462–469.

Frone, M. R., Casey Chosewood, L., Osborne, J. C., & Howard, J. J. (2022). Workplace supported recovery from substance use disorders: Defining the construct, developing a model, and proposing an agenda for future research. *Occupational Health Science, 6*(4), 475–511. https://doi.org/10.1007/s41542-022-00123-x

Garnick, D. W., Horgan, C. M., & Chalk, M. (2006). Performance measures for alcohol and other drug services. *Alcohol Research & Health: The Journal of the National Institute on Alcohol Abuse and Alcoholism, 29*(1), 19–26.

Gaudiano, B. A., Weinstock, L. M., & Miller, I. W. (2011). Improving treatment adherence in patients with bipolar disorder and substance abuse: Rationale and initial development of a novel psychosocial approach. *Journal of Psychiatric Practice, 17*(1), 5–20. https://doi.org/10.1097/01.pra.0000393840.18099.d6

Guyer, J., Traube, A., & Deshchenko, O. (2021). *Speaking the same language: A toolkit for strengthening patient-centered addiction care in the United States.* American Society of Addiction Medicine. https://www.asam.org/asam-criteria/toolkit

Hall, W., Carter, A., & Forlini, C. (2015). The brain disease model of addiction: Is it supported by the evidence and has it delivered on its promises? *The Lancet Psychiatry, 2*(1), 105–110.

Halpern, S., Walls, D. O., Gupta, A., Lustig, A., Weinrieb, R. M., Levine, M. H., & Abt, P. L. (2019). Application of Prescription Drug Monitoring Program to detect underreported controlled substance use in patients evaluated for liver transplant. *American Journal of Transplantation, 19*(12), 3398–3404. https://doi.org/10.1111/ajt.15548

Hasin, D. S., O'Brien, C. P., Auriacombe, M., Borges, G., Bucholz, K., Budney, A., Compton, W. M., Crowley, T., Ling, W., Petry, N. M., Schuckit, M., & Grant, B. F. (2013). DSM-5 criteria for substance use disorders: Recommendations and rationale. *American Journal of Psychiatry, 170*(8), 834–851. https://doi.org/10.1176/appi.ajp.2013.12060782

Hellig, M., MacKillop, J., Martinez, D., Rehm, J., Leggio, L., & Vanderschuren, L. (2021). Addiction as a brain disease revised: Why it still matters, and the need for consilience. *Neuropsychopharmacology, 46*, 1715–1723.

Hingson, R. W., Heeren, T., & Winter, M. R. (2006). Age at drinking onset and alcohol dependence: age at onset, duration, and severity. *Archives of Pediatrics & Adolescent Medicine, 160*(7), 739–746. https://doi.org/10.1001/archpedi.160.7.739

Horton, E. G., Diaz, N., McIlveen, J., Weiner, M., & Mullaney, D. (2010). Mental health and substance use characteristics of flight attendants versus other clients in residential treatment. *Mental Health and Substance Use: Dual Diagnosis, 3*(1), 25–37.

———— (2011). Mental health and substance use characteristics of flight attendants enrolled in an in-patient substance abuse treatment program. *International Journal of Mental Health and Addiction, 9*, 140–150.

Humphreys, K. (2004). *Circles of recovery: Self-help organizations for addictions.* Cambridge University Press.

Insua, D. R., Alfaro, C., Gomez, J., Hernandez-Coronado, P., & Bernal, F. (2019). Forecasting and assessing consequences of aviation safety occurrences. *Safety Science, 111*, 243–252.

Jarvis, M., Williams, J., Hurford, M., Lindsay, D., Lincoln, P., Giles, L., Luongo, P., & Safarian, T. (2017). Appropriate use of drug testing in clinical addiction medicine. *Journal of Addiction Medicine, 11*(3), 163–173. https://doi.org/10.1097/ADM.0000000000000323

Jones, C. M., Baldwin, G. T., Manocchio, T., White, J. O., & Mack, K. A. (2016). Trends in methadone distribution for pain treatment, methadone diversion, and overdose deaths—United States, 2002–2014. *Morbidity and Mortality Weekly Report, 65*(26), 667–671. https://doi.org/10.15585/mmwr.mm6526a2

Jones, C. M., Noonan, R. K., & Compton, W. M. (2020). Prevalence and correlates of ever having a substance use problem and substance use recovery status among adults in the United States, 2018. *Drug and Alcohol Dependence, 214*, 108169. https://doi.org/10.1016/j.drugalcdep.2020.108169

Kadden, R. M., & Litt, M. D. (2011). The role of self-efficacy in the treatment of substance use disorders. *Addictive Behaviors, 36*(12), 1120–1126. https://doi.org/10.1016/j.addbeh.2011.07.032

Kaskutas, L. A. (2009). Alcoholics anonymous effectiveness: Faith meets science. *Journal of Addictive Diseases, 28*(2), 145–157.

Kay, G. & Belanger, H. (2023). *Impairment effects: Pharmacotherapies for alcohol use disorder (AUD) and opioid use disorder (OUD) treatment.* Commissioned paper for the Study and Recommendations on the HIMS, FADAP, and Other Drug and Alcohol Programs within the USDOT. National Academies of Sciences, Engineering, and Medicine. https://nap.nationalacademies.org/resource/27025/Gary_Kay_and_Heather_Balenger_Impairment_Effects_Pharmacotherapies_for_Alcohol_Use_Disorder_and_Opiod_Use_Disorder_commissioned_paper.pdf

Kelly, J. F., & Yeterian, J. D. (2011). The role of mutual-help groups in extending the framework of treatment. *Alcohol Research & Health, 33*(4), 350–355. https://www.ncbi.nlm.nih.gov/pmc/articles/PMC3860535/

Kelly, J. F., Greene, M. C., & Bergman, B. G. (2014). Do drug-dependent patients attending Alcoholics Anonymous rather than Narcotics Anonymous do as well? A Prospective, lagged, matching analysis. *Alcohol and Alcoholism, 49*(6), 645–653. https://doi.org/10.1093/alcalc/agu066

Kelly, J. F., Humphreys, K., & Ferri, M. (2020). Alcoholics Anonymous and other 12-step programs for alcohol use disorder. *The Cochrane Database of Systematic Reviews, 3*(3), CD012880. https://doi.org/10.1002/14651858.CD012880.pub2

Kennedy-Hendricks, A., Barry, C. L., Gollust, S. E., Ensminger, M. E., Chisolm, M. S., & McGinty, E. E. (2017). Social stigma toward persons with prescription opioid use disorder: Associations with public support for punitive and public health-oriented policies. *Psychiatric Services, 68*(5), 462–469. https://doi.org/10.1176/appi.ps.201600056

Klapper, E. S., & Ruff-Stahl, H. J. K. (2019). Effects of the pilot shortage on the regional airline industry: A 2023 forecast. *International Journal of Aviation, Aeronautics, and Aerospace, 6*(3), 2. https://doi.org/10.15394/ijaaa.2019.1321

Lail, P., & Fairbairn, N. (2018). Patients with substance use disorders leaving against medical advice: Strategies for improvement. *Journal of Addiction Medicine, 12*(6), 421–423. https://doi.org/10.1097/ADM.0000000000000432

Lenzer J. (2016). Physician health programs under fire. *BMJ (Clinical Research ed.), 353,* i3568. https://doi.org/10.1136/bmj.i3568

Leshner, A. I. (1997). Addiction is a brain disease, and it matters. *Science, 278*(5335), 45–47. https://doi.org/10.1126/science.278.5335.45

Lewis, R. J., Forster, E. M., Whinnery, J. E., & Webster, N. L. (2014). *Aircraft-assisted pilot suicides in the United States, 2003-2012.* Federal Aviation Administration. https://www.faa.gov/data_research/research/med_humanfacs/oamtechreports/2010s/media/201402.pdf

Lim, S., Cherian, T., Katyal, M., Goldfeld, K. S., McDonald, R., Wiewel, E., Khan, M., Krawczyk, N., Braunstein, S., Murphy, S. M., Jalali, A., Jeng, P. J., MacDonald, R., & Lee, J. D. (2023). Association between jail-based methadone or buprenorphine treatment for opioid use disorder and overdose mortality after release from New York City jails 2011-17. *Addiction, 118*(3). https://doi.org/10.1111/add.16071

Liu, S., Wang, M., Bamberger, P., Shi, J., & Bacharach, S. B. (2015). The dark side of socialization: A longitudinal investigation of newcomer alcohol use. *Academy of Management Journal, 58*(2), 334–355. https://doi.org/10.5465/amj.2013.0239

Manthey, J. S., K., & Rehm, J. (2022). Alcohol and health [Correspondence]. *Lancet, 400*(10365), 1764–1765. https://doi.org/https://doi.org/10.1016/S0140-6736(22)02123-7

Marrow, S., & Coplen, M. (2017). Safety culture: A significant influence on safety in transportation (Rosa P No. 32538). National Transportation Library, Bureau of Transportation Statistics, U.S. Department of Transportation. https://rosap.ntl.bts.gov/view/dot/32538

Mattick, R. P., Breen, C., Kimber, J., & Davoli, M. (2014). Buprenorphine maintenance versus placebo or methadone maintenance for opioid dependence. *The Cochrane Database of Systematic Reviews,* (2), CD002207.

McCarty, D., Braude, L., Lyman, D. R., Dougherty, R. H., Daniels, A. S., Ghose, S. S., & Delphin-Rittmon, M. E. (2014). Substance abuse intensive outpatient programs: Assessing the evidence. *Psychiatric Services, 65*(6), 718–726.

McKay J. R. (2009). Continuing care research: What we have learned and where we are going. *Journal of Substance Abuse Treatment, 36*(2), 131–145. https://doi.org/10.1016/j.jsat.2008.10.004

McKee, D. D., & Chappel, J. N. (1992). Spirituality and medical practice. *The Journal of Family Practice, 35*(2), 205–208. https://cdn.mdedge.com/files/s3fs-public/jfp-archived-issues/1992-volume_34/JFP_1992-08_v35_i2_spirituality-and-medical-practice.pdf

McLellan A. T. (2017). Substance misuse and substance use disorders: Why do they matter in healthcare? *Transactions of the American Clinical and Climatological Association, 128*, 112–130.

McLellan, A. T., Koob, G. F., & Volkow, N. D. (2022). Preaddiction—A missing concept for treating substance use disorders. *JAMA Psychiatry, 79*(8), 749–751. https://doi.org/10.1001/jamapsychiatry.2022.1652

McLellan, A. T., Lewis, D. C., O'Brien, C. P., & Kleber, H. D. (2000). Drug dependence, a chronic medical illness: Implications for treatment, insurance, and outcomes evaluation. *JAMA, 284*(13), 1689–1695. https://doi.org/10.1001/jama.284.13.1689

McLellan, A. T., Skipper, G. S., Campbell, M., & DuPont, R. L. (2008). Five-year outcomes in a cohort study of physicians treated for substance use disorders in the United States. *BMJ, 337*, a2038. https://doi.org/10.1136/bmj.a2038

McPherson, T. L., Goplerud, E., Derr, D., Mickenberg, J., & Courtemanche, S. (2010). Telephonic screening and brief intervention for alcohol misuse among workers contacting the employee assistance program: A feasibility study. *Drug and Alcohol Review, 29*(6), 641–646.

Mee-Lee, D. (2013). *The new ASAM criteria for the treatment of addictive, substance-related, and co-occurring conditions—What you might need to re-form for healthcare reform.* https://dbhdid.ky.gov/dbh/documents/ksaods/2014/Mee-Lee1.pdf

Mee-Lee, D., Shulman, G. D., Fishman, M.J., Gastfriend, D.R., Miller (Eds.). (2013). *The ASAM criteria: Treatment criteria for addictive, substance-related, and co-occurring conditions* (3rd ed.). The Change Companies.

Mello, M. J., Becker, S. J., Bromberg, J., Baird, J., Zonfrillo, M. R., & Spirito, A. (2018). Implementing alcohol misuse SBIRT in a national cohort of pediatric trauma centers—A type III hybrid effectiveness-implementation trial. *Implementation Science, 13*, 35. https://doi.org/10.1186/s13012-018-0725-x

Merlo, L. J., Campbell, M. D., Shea, C., White, W., Skipper, G. E., Sutton, J. A., & DuPont, R. L. (2022). Essential components of physician health program monitoring for substance use disorder: A survey of participants 5 years post successful program completion. *The American Journal on Addictions, 31*(2), 115–122. https://doi.org/10.1111/ajad.13257

Milward, J., Lynskey, M., & Strang, J. (2014). Solving the problem of non-attendance in substance abuse services. *Drug and Alcohol Review, 33*(6), 625–636. https://doi.org/10.1111/dar.12194

Minozzi, S., Amato, L., Vecchi, S., Davoli, M., Kirchmayer, U., & Verster, A. (2011). Oral naltrexone maintenance treatment for opioid dependence. *The Cochrane Database of Systematic Reviews, 2011*(4), CD001333.

Modell, J. G., & Mountz, J. M. (1990). Drinking and flying—the problem of alcohol use by pilots. *The New England Journal of Medicine, 323*(7), 455–461. https://doi.org/10.1056/nejm199008163230706

Monti, P. M., Abrams, D. B., Kadden, R. M., & Cooney, N. L. (1989). *Treating alcohol dependence: A coping skills training guide.* The Guilford Press.

Moos, R. H., Finney, J. W., Ouimette, P. C., & Suchinsky, R. T. (1999). A comparative evaluation of substance abuse treatment: I. Treatment orientation, amount of care, and 1-year outcomes. *Alcoholism, Clinical and Experimental Research, 23*(3), 529–536.

Mrazek, P. J., & Haggerty, R. J. (Eds.). (1994). *Reducing risks for mental disorders: Frontiers for preventive intervention research.* National Academies Press.

Mumenthaler, M., Yesavage, J., Taylor, J., O'Hara, R., Friedman, L., Lee, H., & Kraemer, H. (2003). Psychoactive drugs and pilot performance: A comparison of nicotine, donepezil, and alcohol effects. *Neuropsychopharmacology, 28,* 1366–1373.

Murthy, V. (2016). *Facing addiction in America: The surgeon general's report on alcohol, drugs, and health.* U.S. Department of Health and Human Services.

National Academies of Sciences, Engineering, and Medicine. (2016). *Ending discrimination against people with mental and substance use disorders: The evidence for stigma change.* National Academies Press.

National Highway Traffic Safety Administration. (2000). *A review of the literature on the effects of low doses of alcohol on driving-related skills.* https://one.nhtsa.gov/people/injury/research/pub/hs809028/title.htm

National Institute on Alcohol Abuse and Alcoholism (NIAAA). (n.d.). *What is a "standard drink?" National Institutes of Health, U.S. Department of Health and Human Services.* https://www.rethinkingdrinking.niaaa.nih.gov/how-much-is-too-much/what-counts-as-a-drink/whats-a-standard-drink.aspx

———. (2021). *Alcohol use disorder: A comparison between DSM–IV and DSM–5.* National Institutes of Health, U.S. Department of Health and Human Services. https://www.niaaa.nih.gov/publications/brochures-and-fact-sheets/alcohol-use-disorder-comparison-between-dsm

National Institute on Drug Abuse (NIDA). (n.d.) *Screening and assessment tools chart.* https://nida.nih.gov/nidamed-medical-health-professionals/screening-tools-resources/chart-screening-tools

———. (2007). *Principles of drug addiction treatment: A research based guide* (3rd ed.). https://nida.nih.gov/sites/default/files/675-principles-of-drug-addiction-treatment-a-research-based-guide-third-edition.pdf

National Institute of Mental Health. (n.d.) *Substance use and co-occurring mental disorders. Office of Science Policy, Planning, and Communications.* https://www.nimh.nih.gov/health/topics/substance-use-and-mental-health

National Transportation Safety Board. (2020). *2013–2017 Update to Drug Use Trends in Aviation. Safety Research* (Report No. NTSB/SS-20/01).

Newcomer, K. E., Hatry, H. P., & Wholey, J. S. (Eds.). (2015). *Handbook of practical program evaluation.* Jossey-Bass & Pfeiffer Imprints, Wiley.

Nixon S. J. (1995). Assessing cognitive impairment. *Alcohol Health and Research World, 19*(2), 97–103.

Nordberg, C. (2022). *Analysis of FADAP database.* Commissioned paper for the Study and Recommendations on the HIMS, FADAP, and Other Drug and Alcohol Programs within the USDOT. National Academies of Sciences, Engineering, and Medicine.

O'Connor, L. E., Berry, J. W., Inaba, D., Weiss, J., & Morrison, A. (1994). Shame, guilt, and depression in men and women in recovery from addiction. *Journal of Substance Abuse Treatment, 11*(6), 503–510. https://doi.org/10.1016/0740-5472(94)90001-9

Olsen, E. O., O'Donnell, J., Mattson, C. L., Schier, J. G., & Wilson, N. O. (2019). Notes from the field: Unintentional drug overdose deaths with Kratom detected—27 States, July 2016–December 2017. *Morbidity and Mortality Weekly Report, 68*(14), 326–327. https://doi.org/10.15585/mmwr.mm6814a2

O'Malley, S. S. (1996). Opioid antagonists in the treatment of alcohol dependence: Clinical efficacy and prevention of relapse. *Alcohol and* Alcoholism, *31*(Suppl 1), 77–81. https://www.ncbi.nlm.nih.gov/pubmed/9845042

Picard, E., Aparcero, M., Nijdam-Jones, A., & Rosenfeld, B. (2023). Identifying positive impression management using the MMPI-2 and the MMPI-2-RF: A meta-analysis. *The Clinical Neuropsychologist, 37*(3), 545–561. https://doi.org/10.1080/13854046.2022.2077237

Pinedo, M. (2019). A current re-examination of racial/ethnic disparities in the use of substance abuse treatment: Do disparities persist? *Drug and Alcohol Dependence, 202,* 162–167. https://doi.org/10.1016/j.drugalcdep.2019.05.017

Porges, C.R. (2013). Substance abuse in aviation: Clinical and practical implications. In C. H. Kennedy & F. G. Kay (Eds) *Aeromedical psychology* (pp. 107–123). Ashgate Publishing Limited.

Puchalski, C., Ferrell, B., Virani, R., Otis-Green, S., Baird, P., Bull, J., Chochinov, H., Handzo, G., Nelson-Becker, H., Prince-Paul, M., Pugliese, K., & Sulmasy, D. (2009). Improving the quality of spiritual care as a dimension of palliative care: The report of the Consensus Conference. *Journal of Palliative Medicine, 12*(10), 885–904. https://doi.org/10.1089/jpm.2009.0142

Ren, X., & Foster, D. (2011). Women's experiences of work and family conflict in a Chinese airline. *Asia Pacific Business Review, 17*(3), 325–341.

Richardson, G. E. (2002). The metatheory of resilience and resiliency. *Journal of Clinical Psychology, 58*(3), 307–321. https://doi.org/10.1002/jclp.10020

Roche, A., Kostadinov, V., & Pidd, K. (2019). *The stigma of addiction in the workplace: An essential guide.* Springer.

Schramm-Sapyta, N. L., Walker, Q. D., Caster, J. M., Levin, E. D., & Kuhn, C. M. (2009). Are adolescents more vulnerable to drug addiction than adults? Evidence from animal models. *Psychopharmacology, 206*(1), 1–21. https://doi.org/10.1007/s00213-009-1585-5.

Shaw, M. F., McGovern, M. P., Angres, D. H., & Rawal, P. (2004), Physicians and nurses with substance use disorders. *Journal of Advanced Nursing, 47,* 561–571. https://doi.org/10.1111/j.1365-2648.2004.03133.x

Sheridan, J., & Winkler, H. (1989). Evaluation of drug testing in the workplace. *NIDA Research Monograph, 91,* 195–216.

Shorey, R. C., Brasfield, H., Anderson, S., & Stuart, G. L. (2014). Early maladaptive schemas in a sample of airline pilots seeking residential substance use treatment: An initial investigation. *Mental Health and Substance Use, 7*(1), 73–83. https://doi.org/10.1080/17523281.2013.770414

Skaggs, V., & Norris, A. (2021). *2018 aerospace medical certification statistical handbook.* Civil Aerospace Medical Institute, Federal Aviation Administration. https://rosap.ntl.bts.gov/view/dot/57232

Skinner, M. D., Lahmek, P., Pham, H., & Aubin, H. J. (2014). Disulfiram efficacy in the treatment of alcohol dependence: A meta-analysis. *Public Library of Science One, 9*(2), e87366. https://doi.org/10.1371/journal.pone.0087366

Sliedrecht, W., de Waart, R., Witkiewitz, K., & Roozen, H. G. (2019). Alcohol use disorder relapse factors: A systematic review. *Psychiatry Research, 278,* 97–115.

Snyder, Q. (2021, September 13–September 15). *Welcome and orientation.* 2021 HIMS Advanced Topics Seminar, Denver, CO, USA.

Snyder, Q. (2022, September 11–September 13). *HIMS overview.* 2022 HIMS Basic Education Seminar, Denver, CO, USA.

Squalli, J., & Saad, M. (2006). Accidents airline safety perceptions and consumer demand. *Journal of Economics and Finance, 30*(3), 297–305. https://doi.org/10.1007/BF02752736

Steinhoff, A., Shanahan, L., Bechtiger, L., Zimmermann, J., Ribeaud, D., Eisner, M. P., Baumgartner, M. R., & Quednow, B. B. (2023). When substance use is underreported: Comparing self-reports and hair toxicology in an urban cohort of young adults. *Journal of the American Academy of Child and Adolescent Psychiatry, 62*(7), 791–804. https://doi.org/10.1016/j.jaac.2022.11.011

Strand, T. E., Lystrup, N., & Martinussen, M. (2022). Under-reporting of self-reported medical conditions in aviation: A cross-sectional survey. *Aerospace Medicine and Human Performance, 93*(4), 376–383.

Substance Abuse and Mental Health Services Administration (SAMHSA). (2019a). *A guide to SAMHSA's strategic prevention framework.* U.S. Department of Health and Human Services. https://www.samhsa.gov/sites/default/files/20190620-samhsa-strategic-prevention-framework-guide.pdf

———. (2019b). *Substance use disorders recovery with a focus on employment and education.* Evidence-based resource guide series. U.S. Department of Health and Human Services. https://store.samhsa.gov/sites/default/files/SAMHSA_Digital_Download/pep21-pl-guide-6.pdf

———. (2021). *Key substance use and mental health indicators in the United States: Results from the 2020 National Survey on Drug Use and Health.* U.S. Department of Health and Human Services. https://www.samhsa.gov/data/sites/default/files/reports/rpt35325/NSDUHFFRPDFWHTMLFiles2020/2020NSDUHFFR1PDFW102121.pdf

———. (2022a). *2020 National Survey on Drug Use and Health detailed tables.* U.S. Department of Health and Human Services. https://www.samhsa.gov/data/report/2020-nsduh-detailed-tables

———. (2022b). *Screening, brief intervention, and referral to treatment (SBIRT).* U.S. Department of Health and Human Services. https://www.samhsa.gov/sbirt

Substance Abuse and Mental Health Services Administration & Office of the Surgeon General. (2016). Chapter 6: Health care systems and substance use disorder. *Facing Addiction in America: The Surgeon General's report on alcohol, drugs, and health.* U.S. Department of Health and Human Services.

Substance Abuse Center for Behavioral Health Statistics and Quality. (2023). *2021 National Survey on Drug Use and Health detailed tables.* Substance Abuse and Mental Health Services Administration, U.S. Department of Health and Human Services. https://www.samhsa.gov/data/report/2021-nsduh-detailed-tables

Sudhinaraset, M., Wigglesworth, C., & Takeuchi, D. T. (2016). Social and cultural contexts of alcohol use: Influences in a social-ecological framework. *Alcohol Research: Current Reviews, 38*(1), 35–45.

Sulmasy, D. P. (2002). A biopsychosocial-spiritual model for the care of patients at the end of life. *Gerontologist, 43*(Suppl 3), 24–33. https://doi.org/10.1093/geront/42.suppl_3.24

Suthatorn, P., & Charoensukmongkol, P. (2022). Effects of trust in organizations and trait mindfulness on optimism and perceived stress of flight attendants during the COVID-19 pandemic. *Personnel Review, 52*(3), 882–899. https://doi.org/10.1108/PR-06-2021-0396

Taylor, B. G., Maitra, P., Mumford, E., & Liu, W. (2022). Sexual harassment of law enforcement officers: Findings from a nationally representative survey. *Journal of Interpersonal Violence, 37*(11-12), NP8454–NP8478. https://doi.org/10.1177/0886260520978180

Taranowski, C. & Mahieu, K. (2013). Trends in employee assistance program implementation, structure, and utilization, 2009 to 2010. *Journal of Workplace Behavioral Health, *(28). 172–191. https://doi.org/10.1080/15555240.2013.808068

Troyer, H. L., & Bidaisee, S. (2022). The impact of COVID-19 on the aviation industry: A literature review. *International Public Health Journal, 14*(1), 13–21.

U.S. Preventive Services Task Force, Curry, S. J., Krist, A. H., Owens, D. K., Barry, M. J., Caughey, A. B., Davidson, K. W., Doubeni, C. A., Epling, J. W., Jr, Kemper, A. R., Kubik, M., Landefeld, C. S., Mangione, C. M., Silverstein, M., Simon, M. A., Tseng, C. W., & Wong, J. B. (2018). Screening and behavioral counseling interventions to reduce unhealthy alcohol use in adolescents and adults: US preventive services task force recommendation statement. *Journal of the American Medical Association, 320*(18), 1899–1909.

Vardiman, J. (2008). *Air crew alcohol and drug policies: A survey of FAR of Part 91 corporate/executive flight operations* [Unpublished master's thesis]. University of North Dakota.

Vayr, F., Herin, F., Jullian, B., Soulat, J. M., & Franchitto, N. (2019). Barriers to seeking help for physicians with substance use disorder: A review. *Drug and Alcohol Dependence, 199*, 116–121.

Volkow, N. D., & Koob, G. (2015). Brain disease model of addiction: Why is it so controversial? *Lancet Psychiatry, 2*(8), 677–679. https://doi.org/10.1016/s2215-0366(15)00236-9

Volkow, N. D., Koob, G. F., & McLellan, A. T. (2016). Neurobiologic advances from the brain disease model of addiction. *New England Journal of Medicine, 374*(4), 363–371. https://doi.org/10.1056/NEJMra1511480

Wakeman, S. E. (2017). Medications for addiction treatment: Changing language to improve care. *Journal of Addiction Medicine, 11*(1), 1–2 https://doi.org/10.1097/ADM.0000000000000275

Wakeman, S. E., Larochelle, M. R., Ameli, O., Chaisson, C. E., McPheeters, J. T., Crown, W. H., Azocar, F., & Sanghavi, D. M. (2020). Comparative effectiveness of different treatment pathways for opioid use disorder. *JAMA Network Open, 3*(2), e1920622. https://doi.org/10.1001/jamanetworkopen.2019.20622

Walton, M. T., & Hall, M. T. (2016). The effects of employment interventions on addiction treatment outcomes: A review of the literature. *Journal of Social Work Practice in the Addictions, 6*(4), 358–384, https://doi.org/10.1080/1533256X.2016.1235429

West, S. L., O'Neal, K. K., & Graham, C. W. (2000). A meta-analysis comparing the effectiveness of buprenorphine and methadone. *Journal of Substance Abuse, 12*(4), 405–414.

Westermeyer, J. (2014). Alcoholics anonymous and spiritual recovery: A cultural perspective. *Alcoholism Treatment Quarterly, 32*(2-3), 157–172. https://doi.org/10.1080/07347324.2014.907049

Wisdom, J. (2022). *Call for perspectives and qualitative interview analysis.* Commissioned paper for the Study and Recommendations on the HIMS, FADAP, and Other Drug and Alcohol Programs within the USDOT. National Academies of Sciences, Engineering, and Medicine.

Wooley, C. N., Rogers, R., Fiduccia, C. E., & Kelsey, K. (2013). The effectiveness of substance use measures in the detection of full and partial denial of drug use. *Assessment, 20*(6), 670–680.

World Health Organization (2023). *No level of alcohol consumption is safe for our health.* https://www.who.int/europe/news/item/04-01-2023-no-level-of-alcohol-consumption-is-safe-for-our-health

Wu, A. C., Donnelly-McLay, D., Weisskopf, M. G., McNeely, E., Betancourt, T. S., & Allen, J. G. (2016). Airplane pilot mental health and suicidal thoughts: a cross-sectional descriptive study via anonymous web-based survey. *Environmental Health: A Global Access Science Source, 15*(1), 121.

Xiao, J., Mao, J. Y., & Quan, J. (2022). Flight attendants staying positive! The critical role of career orientation amid the COVID-19 pandemic. *International Journal of Contemporary Hospitality Management, 34*(11), 4312–4328. https://doi.org/10.1108/IJCHM-08-2021-0965

Yang, L. H., Wong, L. Y., Grivel, M. M., & Hasin, D. S. (2017). Stigma and substance use disorders: An international phenomenon. *Current Opinion in Psychiatry, 30*(5), 378–388. https://doi.org/10.1097/yco.0000000000000351

Zschucke, E., Heinz, A., & Ströhle, A. (2012). Exercise and physical activity in the therapy of substance use disorders. *The Scientific World Journal, 2012*, 1–19. https://doi.org/10.1100/2012/901741

Appendix A

Other Alcohol and Drug Programs in the Transportation Sector

This appendix provides a general description of selected other alcohol and drug programs in the non-aviation industry within the U.S. Department of Transportation (DOT). Information covered is limited to the Federal Motor Carrier Safety Administration (FMCSA), Federal Railroad Administration (FRA), and the Federal Transit Administration (FTA) due to their programs providing the most complete and prompt responses to committee inquiries. The discussion highlights the salient characteristics of these drug and alcohol programs based on applicable rules and implementation guidelines under each transportation modal administration. Specific programs established within each administration were not reviewed.

REGULATORY CONTEXT: ALCOHOL AND DRUG PROGRAMS IN THE NON-AVIATION SECTOR

Title V of Public Law 102-143, known as the Omnibus Transportation Employee Testing Act of 1991,[1] mandates that the Secretary of Transportation issue regulations in addressing workplace drug and alcohol misuse by testing employees in safety-sensitive positions. These DOT testing regulations are codified under 49 Code of Federal Regulations (CFR) § 40.[2] The regulations spell out the procedures and requirements on how to conduct the tests, and the activities involving all concerned parties—employers, safety-sensitive transportation employees (including

---

[1] https://www.transportation.gov/odapc/omnibus-transportation-employee-testing-act-1991
[2] https://www.transportation.gov/odapc/part40

self-employed, contractors, and volunteers), and service agents. A positive test result, refusal to test (including adulterating or substituting a urine specimen), and any other violation of the prohibition on the use of alcohol and drugs under DOT regulations require removal of covered employees from safety-sensitive duties.

In addition, under DOT regulations each of the federally regulated transportation administrations has established procedures and implementation guidelines that govern the alcohol and drug misuse programs specific to their workplace operations. The succeeding paragraphs highlight some of the program attributes.

FMCSA

FMCSA is the agency delegated with the authority and responsibility for issuing and implementing rules that address the drug and alcohol misuse in the commercial motor carrier transportation sector. Embodied in 49 CFR § 382, these FMCSA rules are to establish programs designed to help prevent accidents and injuries resulting from the misuse of alcohol or use of controlled substances by drivers of commercial motor vehicles (CMVs).[3]

The employer, a person (including an individual who is self-employed) or entity, has the overall responsibility of implementing the DOT and FMCSA drug and alcohol program requirements. DOT's Office of Drug and Alcohol Policy and Compliance publication,[4] *What Employers Need to Know About DOT Drug and Alcohol Testing [Guidance and Best Practices]*, and FMCSA's publication,[5] *Implementation Guidelines for Alcohol and Drug Regulations*, are key resources for employers in establishing their alcohol and drug programs.

Employers are not the same as service agents:

> A service agent is any person or entity, other than an employee of the motor carrier, used to help implement the DOT and FMCSA drug and alcohol testing regulations. These might include a urine collector, a breath alcohol technician, a screening test technician, a laboratory, a medical review officer, a substance abuse professional (SAP), or a consortium/third-party administrator in charge of coordinating the employer's testing services. Service agents may be used to administer part or all of an employer's DOT drug and alcohol testing program.[6]

---

[3] https://www.ecfr.gov/current/title-49/subtitle-B/chapter-III/subchapter-B/part-382

[4] https://www.transportation.gov/odapc/employer_handbook

[5] https://www.fmcsa.dot.gov/regulations/drug-alcohol-testing/implementation-guidelines-alcohol-and-drug-regulations

[6] https://www.fmcsa.dot.gov/regulations/drug-alcohol-testing/what-are-service-agents

Hiring service agents, however, does not relieve the employer of the oversight responsibility and accountability in carrying out the DOT and FMCSA testing regulations.

Drivers operating CMVs (e.g., trucks and buses), that is, commercial driver license and commercial learners permit holders, perform safety-sensitive functions and are subject to the DOT controlled substance and alcohol testing regulations. A driver is defined in the regulation to include but not limited to full-time, regularly employed drivers; casual, intermittent, or occasional drivers; leased drivers and independent owner-operator contractors. They are holders of commercial driving licenses (CDLs).

Drug and Alcohol Testing

DOT testing involves identifying a blood alcohol concentration of 0.04 or greater, resulting in the removal of the covered employee from performing any safety-sensitive functions until completion of the return to duty process. A driver with a blood alcohol concentration of 0.02 or greater, but less than 0.04, is removed from duty for 24 hours per FMCSA regulation.

FMCSA regulations also require testing in specific CMV accidents (49 CFR § 382.303) resulting in a fatality, bodily injury that requires immediate medical treatment, or one or more motor vehicles requiring to be towed away from the crash site.

FMCSA requires the DOT testing of the five classes of substances: marijuana, cocaine, opiates (opium and codeine derivatives), amphetamines and methamphetamines, and phencyclidine. However, motor carrier employers are not prohibited from instituting a "company authority" testing program (non-DOT program). The non-DOT program is in addition to and distinct from the required DOT testing. This means the employer may test additional substances or may use non-urine specimens but cannot be used in lieu of the DOT requirements.

Referral for Evaluation and Treatment

Drivers of commercial motor vehicles who admit to alcohol misuse or controlled substance use are not subject to the referral, evaluation, and treatment requirements if they meet the conditions specified in 49 CFR § 382.121(a), which include an admission made in accordance with a qualified voluntary self-identification program or policy established by the employer. The voluntary self-identification program or policy must be consistent with 49 CFR § 382.121(b).

Employers are required to refer any driver who has used controlled substances or misused alcohol to a substance abuse professional (SAP) for evaluation regardless of the consequences (e.g., employment termination) specified in the employer's policy. The SAP is required to recommend the appropriate treatment and/or education to a driver who has tested positive on a DOT-controlled substances or alcohol test. However, employers are not required to provide, or to pay for, rehabilitation and treatment programs.[7]

Depending on the SAP's evaluation and recommendation, the following treatment types may be recommended: inpatient setting in a hospital or residential treatment center which includes supervised detoxification, group therapy, etc., and outpatient setting, including intensive outpatient services and outpatient follow-up services.

Return-to-Duty Procedure

FMCSA guidelines remain consistent with the return-to-duty procedure specified in 49 CFR § 40(o). The SAP certifies readiness of the employee to return to duty and fitness to perform safety-sensitive duties.

Program Oversight and Monitoring

Although the FMCSA regulation does not require employers to establish an Employee Assistance Program (EAP) through which most workplace drug and alcohol misuse is managed, the regulations encourage the use of either an internal EAP or external EAP by joining a consortium of small businesses to pool resources to purchase an EAP service for this purpose.

All drug and alcohol violations by commercial driver license and commercial learners permit holders, per DOT testing regulations, are reported in the FMCSA Commercial Clearinghouse. The Clearinghouse is "a secure online database that gives employers, FMCSA, State Driver Licensing Agencies, and State law enforcement personnel real-time information about CDL driver drug and alcohol program violations."[8]

The clearinghouse serves as a multipurpose database depending on the user roles. For example, Medical Review Officers use it to verify test referrals and results; consortia or service agents use it to report drug violations; SAPs use it to verify initial assessment and eligibility to return to duty; state licensing agencies use it to complete the licensing process; employers use it to query the database as part of their pre-employment process, etc. Registration is required to access the database.

A sample of data contained in a monthly report generated by the clearinghouse is given in Figure A-1, reproduced exactly from the original.

---

[7]https://www.fmcsa.dot.gov/regulations/drug-alcohol-testing/implementation-guidelines-alcohol-and-drug-regulations-chapter-8

[8]https://clearinghouse.fmcsa.dot.gov/Resource/Index/Factsheet

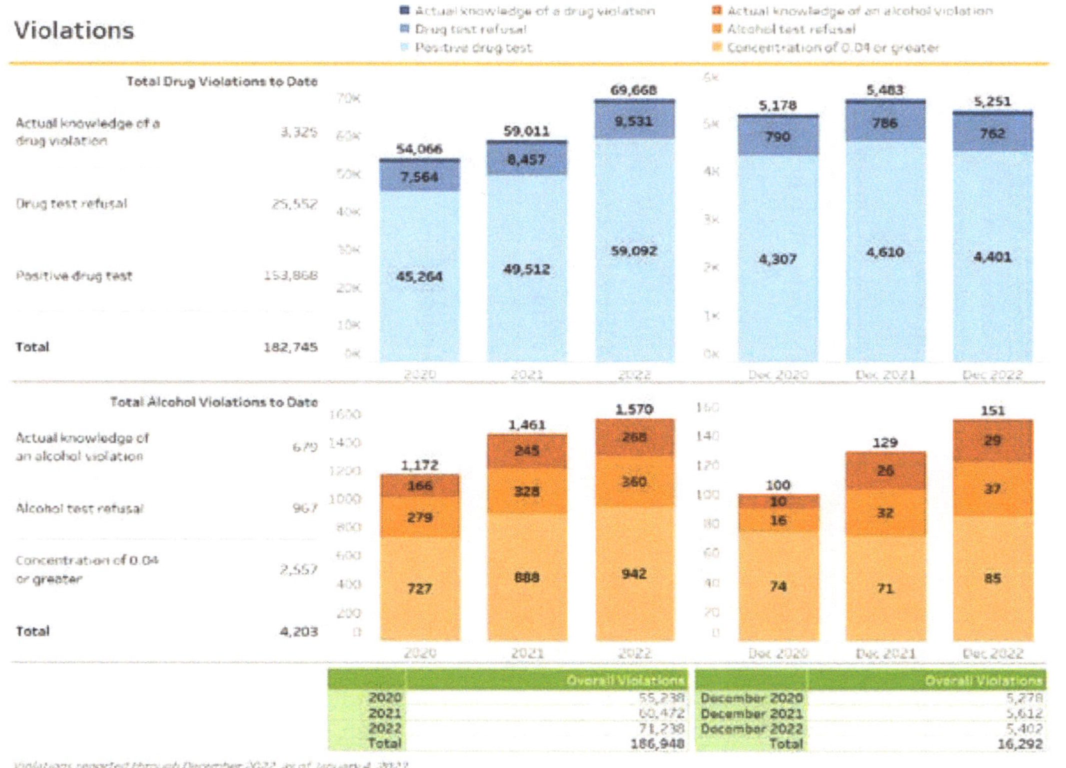

FIGURE A-1 Violations reported to FMCSA clearinghouse since January 6, 2020.
SOURCE: FMCSA Clearinghouse, December 2022 Monthly Summary Report, https://clearinghouse.fmcsa.dot.gov/Resource/Index/monthly-report-Dec2022

FRA

The FRA is the agency delegated with the authority and responsibility for issuing and implementing drug and alcohol misuse rules for inter-city passenger (i.e., Amtrak, commuter) and freight railroad systems of the rail transportation sector. 49 CFR § 219 applies to all railroads and contractors, with noted exceptions made under 49 CFR § 219.3.

Employees, volunteers, and probationary employees performing activities for a railroad or a contractor to a railroad who perform the following regulated services are subject to testing regulations:

- train and engine service (e.g., conductors, brakemen, switchmen, engineers, locomotive hostlers/helpers train service);
- dispatching service/operation (e.g., train dispatchers, control operators);
- signal service who inspects, repair, or maintain signal systems;
- maintenance-of-way employees performing duties of roadway workers as defined in 49 CFR § 214.7; and
- any employee who, on behalf of a railroad, performs mechanical tests or inspections required by 49 CFR § 215, 221, 229, 230, 232, or 238 on railroad rolling equipment, or its components, as defined in "Mechanical or MECH employee" in 49 CFR § 219.5, which became effective March 4, 2022.

Drug and Alcohol Testing

Section 219.101 stipulates that if a test result indicates a blood alcohol concentration below 0.02, the test is negative and is not evidence of alcohol misuse. However, while a federal test result of 0.02 or greater but less than 0.04 is a positive test and may be a violation of a railroad's operating rules, it cannot be used to decertify an engineer under 49 CFR § 240 or a conductor under Part 242. A blood alcohol concentration of 0.04 or greater will affect the certification of the locomotive engineer (49 CFR § 240.119) or conductor (49 CFR § 242.115).

In addition to the five classes of drugs tested under the DOT regulations, FRA also monitors regulated employees' use of prescription and over-the-counter (OTC) drugs. Section 219.103 requires, at a minimum, that a regulated service employee's prescribing physician be made aware of the employee's assigned duties and medical history and deem that the use of that substance (and dosage level) is consistent with the safe performance of the employee's duties. In addition, 49 CFR § 219.103 allows for an employer to require that employees notify the railroad of therapeutic drug use and/or obtain prior approval for such use.[9]

A refusal to test prohibits employees from performing regulated services at any railroad for a minimum of 9 months. Locomotive engineers and conductors will be subject to at least six unannounced drug and alcohol tests during the first 12 months.

Referral for Evaluation and Treatment

Referral for drug and alcohol evaluation and treatment may be coursed through either of the following paths as explained under 49 CFR § 219.1001(k): (a) self-referral, an opportunity given to the employee before the alcohol or drug misuse manifests itself into a detected violation of the rule, or (b) peer-to-peer referral, typically a management-labor partnership that allows an impaired employee to mark-off work, via a 24-hour phone number. Employment relationship with the railroad may be maintained if the covered employee sought assistance through the railroad's voluntary referral program.

Additional referral pathways such as (c) non-peer referral program or (d) alternate programs that meet the specific requirements of 49 CFR § 219.1003 or complying with 49 CFR § 219.1007, or both, may also be made available by a railroad although not guaranteed.

The drug and alcohol counselor (DAC) performs an assessment and clinical evaluation and recommends a course of education and/or treatment facility or program. Treatment recommendations can include inpatient, partial inpatient, outpatient, education programs, and aftercare support services. Education, which may be taken face-to-face or online, may include bona fide drug and alcohol education classes, self-help groups, and community lectures. FRA does not have medical standards apart from aural and visual acuity for certification of locomotive engineers and conductors. A decision to take medication-assisted treatments depends on the DAC's recommendation.

FRA encourages railroads to cover a percentage of the employee's salary to further encourage voluntary self-referrals, but it is based upon the collective bargaining unit and the railroad. In one of the major railroads, for example, referred employees are covered at 80% salary. Otherwise, employees are covered through their company health insurance programs.

---

[9]https://railroads.dot.gov/railroad-safety/divisions/drug-and-alcohol/drug-and-alcohol

Return-to-Duty Procedure

The DAC makes the determination when a covered employee may return to duty. This means successful completion of the DAC's recommended level of care to resolve the employee's identified drug or alcohol abuse problem. Part of the DAC's written notice on the employee's readiness to return to duty consists of requirements for participation in aftercare services such as Alcoholics Anonymous/Narcotics Anonymous meetings and/or therapy. Many Class I rail employees are referred to a treatment provider with a railroad focus.

The employee must have a negative directly observed return-to-duty test, and a minimum of six directly observed follow-up tests in the next 12 months. Follow-up testing programs can last up to 60 months based on the recommended aftercare.

Program Oversight and Monitoring

For monitoring purposes, FRA collects information other than those required by DOT for reporting.[10] The additional information tracks aggregate annual referrals (EAP directed and peer to peer), referral rate, and referral to total violations ratio.

Available data in the past five years are shown below:

TABLE A-1 Drug and Alcohol Referrals, Refusals, and Violations, 2017–2021

Items	2017	2018	2019	2020	2021	Totals
EAP directed and peer-to-peer guided referrals	1,188	1,238	1,797	1,399	1,399	7,021
Drug and alcohol violations + refusals	294	520	531	388	397	2,130
Regulated employees	127,888	133,328	132,196	121,024	121,233	127,134
Referral rate (referrals/ regulated employees)	0.93%	0.93%	1.36%	1.16%	1.15%	1.10%
Referrals to test violations ratio	4.0	2.4	3.4	3.6	3.5	3.3

NOTE: Class I railroad + Amtrak + Commuters.
SOURCE: Jerry Powers presentation, Federal Railroad Administration; Office of Railroad Safety–Office of Railroad Systems, Technology and Innovation, RRS-19, U.S. Department of Transportation.

---

[10]https://www.transportation.gov/odapc/MISreporting

FRA also conducts a triennial audit of the drug and alcohol program, which includes a review of the DAC credentials, referral cases, educational materials, etc. Most recently, FRA started developing a website (currently accessible in a beta version) with interactive dashboards and safety datasets designed to inform citizens, industry, data users, and policy makers.[11]

FTA

FTA is the agency delegated with the authority and responsibility for issuing and implementing drug and alcohol misuse rules for the public mass transportation sector. 49 CFR § 655, in addition to the DOT regulations for drug and alcohol misuse, apply to all FTA employers (recipients and subrecipients of FTA grants) that provide public transportation services, including operators and their contractors.

FTA employers are grantees who receive formula funds through 49 USC § 5307 Urbanized Area Formula (operating and capital), 49 USC § 5309 Transit Capital Investment (capital), 49 USC § 5311 Formula Grants for Rural Areas (operating and capital), or 49 USC § 5339 Buses and Bus Facilities (capital). FTA employers implement the program and conduct testing of their safety sensitive employees. Compliance is a condition to receive financial assistance. On an annual basis, grant recipients are required to certify compliance with 49 CFR § 655 to applicable FTA Regional Office.

The categories of employees with safety-sensitive duties employed by FTA employers and contractors and are covered under the testing regulations, include the following:

- revenue vehicle operation;
- revenue vehicle and equipment maintenance;
- revenue vehicle control/dispatch;
- non-revenue vehicle required to be operated by employees with commercial driver license; and
- armed security personnel.

Drug and Alcohol Testing

Covered employees with blood alcohol concentration of 0.04 or greater or who refuse to submit to testing are prohibited to perform safety-sensitive functions. The employer is required to advise the employee of available resources for evaluating and resolving their alcohol and drug problems.

---

[11] https://railroads.dot.gov/safety-data/accident-and-incident-reporting/accidentincident-dashboards-data-downloads

This includes giving the names, addresses, and telephone numbers of SAPs and counseling and treatment programs.

As specified in 49 CFR § 655.35, an employee with a blood alcohol concentration of at least 0.02 but below 0.04 is prohibited to perform or continue to perform safety-sensitive duties. An employer may choose to permit a retest within eight hours of an alcohol test for confirmation. The covered employee may perform safety sensitive functions only until:

1. The employee's alcohol concentration measures less than 0.02; or
2. The start of the employee's next regularly scheduled duty period, but not less than eight hours following administration of the test.

Employers are not prohibited from adopting a drug-free workplace act or testing substances in addition to the five classes of substance under the DOT regulations. FTA employers may include prescription drugs and OTC drugs in their policy (encouraged). Starting January 18, 2022, four semi-synthetic opioids (hydrocodone, oxycodone, hydromorphone, and oxymorphone) were added while removing MDEA, an amphetamine similar to ecstasy, from the substance test panel. Covered employees may be tested any time before, during, and after performing safety-sensitive duties. 49 CFR § 655.44 of FTA regulations also require post-accident testing.

Referral for Evaluation and Treatment

Only company officials who are in contact with covered employees are authorized to make referrals. This includes dispatchers, street supervisors, and maintenance supervisors. Other employees who are not authorized should know who to contact and be able to substantiate a reasonable suspicion. Only one trained company official is sufficient to refer a covered employee for reasonable-suspicion testing.

Transit employer's EAP serve an important role in FTA's drug and alcohol testing program, particularly for self-referrals.

While FTA regulations require employers to comply with the DOT testing regulations, they are not required to provide or pay for rehabilitation and treatment programs. Two types of treatment are provided: inpatient and outpatient services. They include intensive inpatient (hospital or residential facility), intensive outpatient, and outpatient follow-up services. The SAP develop a treatment program that meets the needs of the employee.

Return-to-Duty Procedure

The return-to-duty procedures in 49 CFR § 40 is followed before an employee is allowed to perform safety-sensitive functions. Pursuant to

49 CFR § 40(o), employers are required to conduct follow-up testing of covered employees upon return to duty.

Program Oversight and Monitoring

FTA maintains an online management information system called DAMIS[12] for drug and alcohol test data reporting. It is accessible only to grantees, states department of transportation, covered employees, contractors, and subrecipients.

SUMMARY

Given adequate time, a more in-depth analysis of the various models of drug and alcohol programs implemented across the transportation modal administrations would be helpful in determining the overall effectiveness of U.S. DOT efforts in addressing drug and alcohol impairment in transportation. From the foregoing discussions, the following program features are likewise underscored for consideration:

1. *Financial support*: FRA's practice of encouraging employers to cover a certain percentage of treatment cost and/or salary of covered employees may motivate covered employees to change their treatment-seeking behavior for early intervention.
2. *Increased panel of substances tested*: Both FRA and FTA had identified the impairment effects of prescription and OTC drugs in the conduct of safety-sensitive functions. They are testing for them in addition to the panel of substances covered under the DOT regulations.
3. *Voluntary referral*: FRA has a specific section requiring railroads to establish self-referral and peer-to-peer referral programs. While voluntary referral may be offered by employers of other modal administrations, they are only encouraged but not required.
4. *Online reporting and monitoring*: While all modal administrations offer some variations of online test result reporting and monitoring, each system shows weaknesses and strengths. An examination of each may help strengthen the reporting system for oversight and decision support. The FMCSA Clearinghouse, for example, is a system developed for different users with varied purposes.
5. *Organized program management*: Standardizing program implementation ensures that availability, accessibility, and equity in treatment is achieved. A national oversight of the drug and alcohol

---

[12]https://transit-safety.fta.dot.gov/DrugAndAlcohol/DAMIS/default.aspx

programs within each administration could minimize variations. For example, FAA has established a national oversight by setting aside funds for this purpose.

6. *Inclusion of mental health evaluation and/or focus on co-occurring mental health and substance use disorders*: Specific rules and regulations reviewed in this appendix have not specifically addressed the issue on mental health. It warrants attention and inclusion in existing regulations, rules, and procedures due to its confounding effects on impairment.

7. *Use of poly-substances*: Similar to the mental health issue, poly-substance use and its impact on impairment should be addressed in the existing regulations, rules, and procedures. Poly-substance use impacts the duration and extent of impairment and thus the return-to-duty criteria may even need to be revisited.

Appendix B

Speakers, Papers, and Literature Review—Data Gathering

June 30, 2022

The lead liaison staff from the Federal Aviation Administration (FAA): **Penny Giovanetti,** Office of Aerospace Medicine; **Tom Cuddy,** Systems and Policy Analysis Division; and **Phil Putter,** Office of Aviation Policy and Plans. These speakers gave an overview of their priorities.

Quay Snyder, program manager of the Human Intervention and Motivational Study (HIMS). Provided an overview of HIMS.

Heather Healy, manager of the Flight Attendant Drug and Alcohol Program (FADAP). Provided an overview of FADAP.

August 22, 2022

Nora Volkow, director of the National Institute on Drug Abuse and a recognized expert on addictions and their treatment.

Thomas McLellan, former deputy director of the Office of National Drug Control Policy, editor of the *Surgeon General's Report on Alcohol and Drugs* (HHS, 2016), and lead researcher on an evaluation of 16 physician health programs that serve physicians with substance abuse disorders (McLellan et al., 2008).

Ted Trippi, legislative assistant for U.S. Senator Jeanne Shaheen of New Hampshire. Provided background on the study's origins and congressional expectations.

November 1, 2022

Gary Kay, chief scientific officer, Cognitive Research Corporation. Gave a presentation, related to his commissioned paper, on aviation issues around impairment, cognition, and treatment.

Sarah Polk, SkyWest Airlines; and Dave St. Hilaire, Allegiant Airlines. Presented the flight attendants' perspective, as both are active in their respective FADAP organizations.

Captain Dave Fielding, British Airways. Gave a presentation on pilot well-being and peer support systems and offered an international perspective.

Andrew LeBovidge, executive vice president, National Air Traffic Controllers Association; **Pat Moy,** manager of drug abatement and regulatory compliance, United Airlines; and **Kip Bowen,** senior manager, Employee Assistance Program, United Airlines. All participated in a panel assessing existing support systems across aviation.

COMMISSIONED AUTHORS AND THEIR PAPERS

The papers listed here were all commissioned for the Study and Recommendations on the HIMS, FADAP, and Other Drug and Alcohol Programs within the U.S. Department of Transportation (DOT) by the Board on Behavioral, Cognitive, and Sensory Sciences, National Academies of Sciences, Engineering, and Medicine, Washington, DC.[1]

Gary Kay and Heather Belanger

Commissioned paper: *Impairment Effects: Pharmacotherapies for Alcohol Use Disorder (AUD) and Opioid Use Disorder (OUD) Treatment* (2022)

Cara Nordberg

Commissioned paper: *Analysis of FADAP Database* (2022)

Jennifer Wisdom

Commissioned paper: *Call for Perspectives and Qualitative Interview Analysis* (2022)

---

[1] See the commissioned paper tab at https://nap.nationalacademies.org/catalog/27025/substance-misuse-programs-in-commercial-aviation-safety-first

MATERIALS REVIEWED FOR LITERATURE SEARCH

The National Academies of Sciences Research Center compiled two literature reviews for the study. The first focused on whether any previous research existed on HIMS and FADAP, along with material describing the structure or effectiveness of other substance-abuse-related programs (non-HIMS/FADAP) within the FAA or DOT.[2] The second examined the wider mental health and well-being of pilots, flight attendants, and other transportation industry employees.

---

[2]Additional information for Appendix A was provided by **Jerry Powers,** Office of Railroad Safety, Federal Railroad Administration; **Iyon Rosario,** Office of Safety & Oversight, Federal Transit Administration; and **Bryan Price,** Drug & Alcohol Program Division, Federal Motor Carriers Safety Administration.

Appendix C

Communications Between the Committee and the Federal Aviation Administration, Human Intervention and Motivational Study, Airline Pilots Association, International, and Congressional Staff

During the course of its work, the committee reached out to the Federal Aviation Administration (FAA), the staff of the Human Intervention and Motivational Study (HIMS), the Airline Pilots Association, International (ALPA), and the Office of U.S. Senator Jeanne Shaheen (the lead Congressional sponsor for the National Academies study). The committee sent requests for data and requests for potential speakers at the workshop or to present to the committee. This appendix details the timing of those committee communications with the various offices for data, lists the information requested by the committee that was not provided by the various offices, and states the rationale for that decision if it was provided to the National Academy of Sciences (NAS).

Date	NAS-FAA Interaction	NAS-HIMS Interaction	NAS-ALPA Interaction	NAS-Shaheen's Office Interaction	Related Outcome(s) (if any)
April 27, 2022		HIMS Program Manager initially offered to share queries and results from the HIMS database and set up a confidentiality data-sharing agreement.			No response provided to NAS.
September 2022		Project staff and committee members attended the annual HIMS Basic Education Seminar in September 2022 to learn about how the program operates. Subsequently, the committee sought to obtain more detailed descriptions of the program experience from the general pilot population.			
October 25, 2022			Draft workshop agenda sent to ALPA, including names of invited pilots chosen by the committee for their expertise.		ALPA provided alternative pilots in current leadership positions.

Date	NAS-FAA Interaction	NAS-HIMS Interaction	NAS-ALPA Interaction	NAS-Shaheen's Office Interaction	Related Outcome(s) (if any)
October 26-31, 2022			NAS-invited pilots decommit to present at workshop.		ALPA senior leadership cited those without direct HIMS expertise should not present.
November 3, 2022		Committee requested data from the FAA-funded HIMS database.			The HIMS Advisory Board denied access, asserting the contract with the FAA and concerns over confidentiality and data disclosure might erode program integrity.
November 3, 2022	The committee requested a copy of the FAA-APLA contract.				No immediate response provided to NAS.
November 7, 2022		Committee created a "Call for Perspectives" tool for gathering lived experiences and requested that HIMS and FADAP officials distribute through their internal networks for confidential submission of data.			The committee received a total of 1,200 responses; 4 were from pilots.

continued

Date	NAS-FAA Interaction	NAS-HIMS Interaction	NAS-ALPA Interaction	NAS-Shaheen's Office Interaction	Related Outcome(s) (if any)
November 9, 2022			The committee again requested access to the HIMS database.		ALPA asserted the contract with HIMS restricted access to the database.
December 2, 2022			The committee requested custom language so that ALPA could run queries by their staff to assuage possible confidentiality concerns.		ALPA asserted sophisticated searches may not result in accurate or reliable results. No data was received.
December 6, 2022				Committee was informed that Senator Shaheen's staff contacted ALPA representatives to allow the committee access to HIMS data.	ALPA asserted that lack of standardized data might lead to inaccurate results and negatively affect analysis.
December 14, 2022	The committee and Senator Shaheen's office requested copy of the contract between FAA and HIMS.				Copy of the contract was delivered to NAS.

Date	NAS-FAA Interaction	NAS-HIMS Interaction	NAS-ALPA Interaction	NAS-Shaheen's Office Interaction	Related Outcome(s) (if any)
December 15, 2022	After review of the contract, the committee noted that the FAA owned the data, not ALPA, and indicated that access to the data would assist the National Academies to fulfill the congressional mandate.				
December 21, 2022	FAA noted that full access would not be provided, rather they offered to provide aggregate data related to HIMS.				No immediate response provided to NAS.
January 30, 2023	The committee asserted its request for HIMS data.				Data was not received by NAS.

Date	NAS-FAA Interaction	NAS-HIMS Interaction	NAS-ALPA Interaction	NAS-Shaheen's Office Interaction	Related Outcome(s) (if any)
February 3, 2023				Senator Shaheen's staff noted the lack of cooperation and access to the data and would inform future possible actions with regard to the HIMS database.	No data received by NAS.

Appendix D

Committee Member Biosketches

RICHARD G. FRANK (*Chair*, he/him) is the Margaret T. Morris Professor of Health Economics emeritus at Harvard Medical School. He is a senior fellow in economic studies and director of the Schaeffer Initiative on Health Policy at the Brookings Institution. Frank previously served as the Deputy Assistant Secretary for Planning and Evaluation at the Department of Health and Human Services directing the office of Disability, Aging and Long-Term Care Policy. Frank's research is focused on the economics of mental health and substance abuse care, long term care financing policy, prescription drug markets, and disability policy. He is co-author with Sherry Glied of the book *Better But Not Well*. Frank received his PhD in economics from Boston University and BA in economics from Bard College.

DAVID L. ALBRIGHT (he/him) is a University Distinguished Research Professor and the Hill Crest Foundation Endowed Chair in Mental Health Research at The University of Alabama. He uses behavioral health and social care expertise across Alabama, serving as principal investigator for multiple state-focused projects that strive to study and improve services, policies, and social conditions for those with mental health, substance use disorder, and trauma-related challenges. Albright is an elected fellow of the American Academy of Social Work and Social Welfare and the National Academies of Practice in Social Work. His research examines both the health status and risk behaviors of individuals with trauma, psychiatric, or substance use history, and barriers and facilitators to their access and utilization of mental health and addiction treatment services. Albright received his MSW and PhD in social work from Florida State University.

DANIEL N. DaSILVA (he/him) is an aerospace and pediatric neuro-psychologist and a partner at the Morris Psychological Group in Parsippany, New Jersey. He is also a part-time lecturer at Rutgers University, Graduate School of Education and he is on staff at Morristown and Overlook Medical Centers in New Jersey. In his practice, DaSilva performs neuropsychological and psychological assessments of aircrew and air traffic controllers. He serves as a neuropsychology consultant to the Federal Air Surgeon of the Federal Aviation Administration and is an external consultant for several major airlines. DaSilva has been deemed qualified by the National Trans-portation Safety Board to provide expert testimony in aviation neuro-psychology. He is a member of the National Academy of Neuropsychology, American Psychological Association, New Jersey Psychological Associa-tion, Aerospace Medical Association, and the Aerospace Human Factors Association. He completed specialized neuropsychology training through the Veteran's Administration in consortium with University Hospital in Newark, New Jersey. He is the 2022 recipient of the Distinguished Service to Neuropsychology award from the American Board of Professional Neuro-psychology. He earned a BA in psychology from Boston College, a MA in counseling psychology from University of Massachusetts at Boston, and a PhD in clinical psychology from Fairleigh Dickinson University.

ROBYN L. HACKER (she/her) is an assistant professor in the Division of Addiction Science, Prevention and Treatment in the Department of Psychiatry at the University of Colorado and the lead psychologist for The Professionals Program at the Center for Dependency Addiction and Rehabilitation where she evaluates and treats professionals in safety sensi-tive occupations. Her clinical work and research interests focus at the inter-sect of substance use disorders, trauma, and co-occurring disorders. Hacker is a licensed psychologist, licensed addiction counselor, and eye movement desensitization and reprocessing consultant. She has worked with youth, adults, and families in residential, intensive outpatient, and standard out-patient settings and has extensive experience treating professional and forensic patients and educating others about mental illness and recovery. Hacker's dissertation project focused on developing and evaluating an online mental health training for law enforcement received the Outstand-ing Dissertation Award from Division 18 of the American Psychological Association. She completed BS degrees in criminal justice and psychology at Loyola University Chicago, a PhD in counseling psychology at Arizona State University, and pre- and post-doctoral fellowships in forensic addic-tion psychology at Yale School of Medicine.

JERMAINE D. JONES (he/him) is an associate professor with the Division on Substance Use Disorders at Columbia University Irving Medical Center.

As faculty, his area of focus has been to better understand how genetic factors influence the risk of developing substance use disorders, and the effectiveness of novel medications. More recently, Jones' research has begun to focus on community-based efforts to reduce the harms associated with opioid and psychostimulant use. Jones' research has been funded by the National Institute on Drug Abuse, Merck Pharmaceuticals, Peter McManus Charitable Trust, and the Gray Matters Benefit of Columbia University. He has served on several National Institutes of Health scientific review committees and is currently on the Board of Directors of the College on Problems of Drug Dependence and the Board of Scientific Affairs of the American Psychological Association. Jones received his PhD in behavioral neuroscience from American University, where his research focused on understanding the abuse potential of cocaine and alcohol. He completed his post-doctoral fellowship with Columbia's Division on Substance Use Disorders researching the pharmacological and neurobiological drivers of opioid use.

MADELINE H. MEIER (she/her) is associate professor in the Department of Psychology at Arizona State University. Her research involves investigation of the causes, courses, and consequences of problematic substance use. Her work documenting the mental health, cognitive, brain, academic, social, economic, and physical health consequences of cannabis use is used regularly by policy makers, public interest groups, psychologists, and physicians. Meier has provided testimony to the U.S. Senate on cannabis effects on health. She is the recipient of the Rising Star Award from the Association for Psychological Science and the Enoch Gordis Award from the Research Society on Alcoholism. Meier received her PhD in psychology from the University of Missouri, completed her clinical psychology internship at the Durham Veterans Affairs Medical Center, and completed her postdoctoral training at Duke University.

MICHELLE N. MEYER (she/her) is an associate professor and chair of the Department of Bioethics & Decision Sciences at Geisinger, where she is also chief bioethics officer and faculty co-director of the Behavioral Insights Team, which uses principles of behavioral science to "nudge" patients, members, and clinicians to make healthy choices. Her normative and empirical research on topics including research ethics and data sharing focuses on the intersection of applied ethics and behavioral science and has been published in leading journals and popular media outlets. Meyer has served on an American Psychological Association blue ribbon commission and serves on the editorial board of *Advances in Methods and Practices in Psychological Science*. She earned a PhD in religious studies with a focus on applied ethics from the University of Virginia and a JD from Harvard Law School, where she was an editor of the Harvard Law Review. Following law school, she clerked for Judge Stanley Marcus of the U.S. Court of Appeals for the Eleventh Circuit.

TERRIE E. MOFFITT (she/her) has extensive expertise in the areas of lifelong aging, mental health, and longitudinal research. She is the associate director of the Dunedin Longitudinal Study, which follows a 1972 birth cohort in New Zealand. She also founded the Environmental Risk Longitudinal Twin Study (E-Risk), which follows a 1994 birth cohort in Britain. Moffitt is a licensed clinical psychologist, an elected fellow of the U.S. National Academy of Medicine, American Academy of Arts and Sciences, British Academy, U.K. Academy of Medical Sciences, and Association of Psychological Science. She is chair of the National Academies of Sciences, Engineering, and Medicine's Board on Behavioral, Cognitive, and Sensory Sciences. Moffitt received her PhD in psychology at the University of Southern California and completed her postdoctoral training at the UCLA Neuropsychiatric Institute.

KATHRYN E. NEWCOMER (she/her) is a professor in the Trachtenberg School of Public Policy and Public Administration at George Washington University, where she has also served as the Trachtenberg School director. She is a fellow of the National Academy of Public Administration and serves on the Comptroller General's Educators' Advisory Panel. She served as president of the American Evaluation Association and president of the Network of the Association of Schools of Public Policy, Affairs and Administration. Newcomer routinely conducts evaluations for federal and local government agencies and nonprofit organizations. She has served on six Committees of the National Academy of Sciences, published 10 books, and written many articles in esteemed journals. Newcomer received her PhD in political science at the University of Iowa.

BERNADETTE E. PHELAN (she/her) has combined executive and senior management experience encompassing the areas of public mental health and substance use services delivery systems, transportation, professional health regulation, and economic development. She has occupied varied positions with a broad range of responsibilities ranging from project director of the Behavioral Health Services Information System administered by the Substance Abuse and Mental Health Services Administration, assistant director for the Arizona Medical Board, chief of research and evaluation for the Division of Behavioral Health Services within the Arizona Department of Health Services, director of Special Studies for the non-profit National Association of State Mental Health Program Directors Research Institute, and a Senior Research Project Manager at Arizona Department of Transportation. Phelan is currently a member of the National Academies of

Sciences, Engineering, and Medicine Transportation Research Board's Committee on Impairment in Transportation and the Committee on Women and Gender in Transportation. She is on the advisory panel for a number of national studies conducted under the National Cooperative Highway Research Program and the Behavioral Traffic Safety Cooperative Research Program. Phelan received her PhD in economics at Keio University and her MA at the University of the Philippines.

JEFFREY SELZER (he/him) is a psychiatrist who specializes in physician and medical student mental health and in addiction treatment. In his work as Medical Director of the Committee for Physician Health, New York's physician health program, he provides direction and oversight for a non-disciplinary pathway for New York physicians and medical students to receive mental health treatment and monitoring. In his work for Northwell Health, he provides direct mental health care to physicians and medical students in the Northwell system. His research experience includes membership in the NIDA Clinical Trials Network (CTN) and service to the CTN as a member of the Executive Committee and Chair of the Research Utilization Committee. Selzer is chair of the Public Policy Committee for the American Society of Addiction Medicine and chair of the Addiction Psychiatry Committee for the New York State Psychiatric Association. He completed a residency in psychiatry at the University of California at Los Angeles and is board certified in psychiatry and in addiction medicine.

MO WANG (he/him) is the Lanzillotti-McKethan Eminent Scholar Chair and the associate dean for Research at the Warrington College of Business at University of Florida. He is also the chair of the Management Department and the director of Human Resource Research Center at University of Florida and is currently serving on the President-track for Society for Industrial-Organizational Psychology. He specializes in research areas of occupational health psychology and human resource management, especially on alcohol use at workplace. He received numerous research awards for his research in these areas. He is an elected Foreign Member of Academia Europaea; he is also a fellow of Academy of Management, the American Psychological Association, the Association for Psychological Science, and the Society for Industrial-Organizational Psychology. Wang was the president of the Society for Occupational Health Psychology. Wang received his PhD from Bowling Green State University.

Appendix E

Disclosure of Unavoidable Conflict of Interest

The conflict-of-interest policy of the National Academies of Sciences, Engineering, and Medicine (http://www.nationalacademies.org/coi) prohibits the appointment of an individual to a committee authoring a Consensus Study Report if the individual has a conflict of interest that is relevant to the task to be performed. An exception to this prohibition is permitted if the National Academies determines that the conflict is unavoidable and the conflict is publicly disclosed. A determination of a conflict of interest for an individual is not an assessment of that individual's actual behavior or character or ability to act objectively despite the conflicting interest.

Daniel DaSilva has a conflict of interest in relation to his service on the Study and Recommendations on the Human Intervention Motivational Study (HIMS), Flight Attendant Drug and Alcohol Program, and Other Drug and Alcohol Programs within the U.S. Department of Transportation Committee because he is an aviation neuropsychologist for a practice that evaluates patients in HIMS.

The National Academies has concluded that in order for the committee to accomplish the tasks for which it was established, its membership must include at least one person who has substantial and direct current expertise treating substance abuse in the aviation industry in order to adequately assess the programs. As described in his biographical summary, DaSilva has extensive current expertise with HIMS in clinical and aviation psychology, including conducting neuropsychological and psychological assessments of pilots and air traffic controllers, as well as patients experiencing acquired injuries, illnesses, psychological disorders, and substance abuse problems.

The National Academies has determined that the experience and expertise of DaSilva is needed for the committee to accomplish the task for which it has been established. The National Academies could not find another available individual with the equivalent experience and expertise who does not have a conflict of interest. Therefore, the National Academies has concluded that the conflict is unavoidable.

The National Academies believes that DaSilva can serve effectively as a member of the committee, and the committee can produce an objective report, taking into account the composition of the committee, the work to be performed, and the procedures to be followed in completing the study.